Autoimmunity

Autoimmunity

Edited by

Andrzej Górski

Hubert Krotkiewski

and

Michał Zimecki

Ludwik Hirszfeld Institute of Immunology and Experimental Therapy,
Polish Academy of Sciences, Wrocław, Poland

KLUWER ACADEMIC PUBLISHERS
DORDRECHT / BOSTON / LONDON

A C.I.P. Catalogue record for this book is available from the Library of Congress.

ISBN 1-4020-0037-5

Published by Kluwer Academic Publishers,
P.O. Box 17, 3300 AA Dordrecht, The Netherlands.

Sold and distributed in North, Central and South America
by Kluwer Academic Publishers,
101 Philip Drive, Norwell, MA 02061, U.S.A.

In all other countries, sold and distributed
by Kluwer Academic Publishers,
P.O. Box 322, 3300 AH Dordrecht, The Netherlands.

Printed on acid-free paper

Printed in the Netherlands.

TABLE OF CONTENTS

PREFACE

The immune system has evolved mechanisms enabling it to discriminate between self and non-self constituents. A normally functioning organism is naturally unresponsive to self antigens originating from clonal deletion, anergy, or an active suppression of self-reactive T cells. The wide spectrum of autoimmune responses may be divided into systemic and organ-specific diseases and encompasses the actions of autoantibodies, autoantigen-autoantibody complexes, and sensitized T lymphocytes.

The aim of this book is to review the current understanding, concepts and hypotheses regarding the pathogenesis and therapeutic approaches in autoimmune disorders. The first six articles are generally concerned with the mechanisms operating in autoimmune phenomena, whereas the subsequent reviews discuss particular phenomena in representative autoimmune diseases.

The introductory article underlines the significance of the interactions between antigen-specific T cells and other elements of the immune system and proposes that not suppression, but rather activation of the immune system, leading to a redirection of the immune response, would be therapeutically beneficial. The next articles present the importance of costimulatory signals in determining various types of immune responses, including autoimmunity, and the role of regulatory T cells. Further, an interesting phenomenon of epitope spreading as a mechanism for the progression of autoimmune diseases is presented. In the following articles, the role of intracellular signaling involving NF-κB in a mouse model of type-1 diabetes is discussed and the involvement of complement regulatory proteins in autoimmunity is evaluated, suggesting their beneficial role in the protection of cells against destructive complement action. The following articles are devoted to a model of experimental autoimmune encephalomyelitis, providing evidence that Fas and FasL contribute to the pathogenesis of the disease and critically reviewing the roles of the relevant cytokines in the model. Subsequent articles are related to the involvement of apoptosis in tissue destruction in the mouse model of Sjögren's syndrome and the mechanisms leading to type-1 diabetes in non-obese diabetic mice. The two final reviews describe the consequence of defects in the functioning of the endocrine-immune axis in the pathophysiology of rheumatoid arthritis and the T cell abnormalities found in this disease.

THE PARADIGMS OF CAUSALITY AND TREATMENT FOR AUTOIMMUNE DISEASE

IRUN R. COHEN

Department of Immunology, Weizmann Institute of Science, Rehovot 76100, Israel

Abstract A key concept in medicine is that rational therapy rests on accurate diagnosis; quite simply, therapy that is not tuned to the cause of the disease will not cure the patient. This does not mean that effective treatments cannot emerge from faulty diagnoses. In truth, much of our therapeutic ensemble is composed of drugs developed as a result of chance observation, random screening, intuition or pre-scientific tradition. Nevertheless, the way to effective therapy is best paved by understanding. Effects are inherent in their causes, so if we want to cure autoimmune diseases using the scientific method, we are obliged to inquire into their causes. By reducing the discordant complexity of the disease to the single cause that underlies it, we can hope to learn the most efficient way to manipulate the disease process. How do we identify a cause when we see one? Quite simply, a single cause is that which is both necessary and sufficient to produce the effect. Here, I explore the general paradigm of autoimmune causality, using multiple sclerosis as a specific example.

Key words: autoimmune disease; therapy; causality; multiple sclerosis; diabetes.

1. GENES OR ENVIRONMENT

Single causes in biology are sought in either of two domains: the genes that program the body and the environment in which the body operates. Health is perceived to be the outcome of a harmonious interaction between one's genome and one's environment, disease the outcome of their discord (Cohen, 2000). Thus, we would like to be able to attribute multiple sclerosis (MS) either to a single faulty gene or to a defined pathogenic agent or stress striking the body from the surroundings. Such is the prevailing paradigm.

Therefore, we are frustrated to learn that MS patients, like persons suffering from other autoimmune diseases, cannot be distinguished from those free of MS by any single gene (Vyse and Todd, 1996). Certainly, there is an HLA--associated genetic predisposition to MS (Oksenbeg et al., 1993b), but the

A. Górski et al. (eds.), Autoimmunity, 1–10.

great majority of people bearing susceptibility genes for MS, or for any other autoimmune disease, will never contract the disease. HLA genes can only tell us who may be susceptible to developing MS, not who is surely going to get MS. In other words, autoimmune diseases cannot be reduced to a gene in the way that sickle cell anemia can be reduced to a gene for hemoglobin S (Gill et al., 1995). Indeed, individuals born with the same genome, i.e. monozygotic twins, have a concordance rate for MS of only about 30% (Ebers et al., 1986). This fact suggests that a factor in the environment must be critical.

However, the development of MS cannot be attributed to a single defined pathogenic agent or environmental circumstance. Viruses, toxins and stresses have all been implicated in certain individuals, but no preceding environmental influence can distinguish as a class all of those suffering from MS from those without MS. MS as a category cannot be reduced to an agent or an agency in the way that hepatitis can be reduced to a virus.

Note, parenthetically, that certain autoimmune diseases can be triggered by infection with specific bacteria, such as group A streptococci, which can induce acute rheumatic fever (Bronze and Dale, 1996). But even in this example, the majority of those infected with the necessary *Streptococcus* do not develop acute rheumatic fever. Certain viruses, such as HIV or hepatitis viruses, may induce autoimmune pathology with more regularity. An MS virus may yet emerge, but at present, MS cannot be reduced to a single underlying element residing in either the genes or in the environment. Must we conclude that MS has no definable cause? Is MS a matter of bad luck only?

2. FORBIDDEN CLONES

Causality implies order: a predictable effect is inherent in a defined cause (Cohen, 2000). Causes, however, can still be random, e.g. mutations.

Obviously, it makes sense to try and reduce the development of an autoimmune disease to a renegade clone of autoimmune lymphocytes, the "forbidden clone" of the classical clonal selection paradigm (Burnet, 1969). Clonal selection assumed that any autoimmune lymphocyte would be deleted automatically; hence, autoimmune diseases would have to be accounted for by a somatic mutation giving rise to an autoimmune clone after the critical period of development during which autoimmune lymphocytes are purged from the immune repertoire. This idea is still being taught. The idea is that the immediate cause, both necessary and sufficient for autoimmune disease, is a clone of autoimmune T or B cells. The autoimmune clone might arise in different persons by different accidents, but once it has arisen, the clone is the cause of disease (Ben-Nun and Cohen, 1982a). In other words, the clone is caused by an accident, the disease by the clone. Conceptually, this would put MS in a class with cancer; a transformed cell is the single cause of the tumor, although the transformed cell itself can be generated by accident.

The question then is whether a single population of specifically autoimmune T cells suffices to cause the complex manifestations of an autoimmune disease. This question motivated my colleagues and me to isolate pure cultures of autoreactive T cells *in vitro* and study their effects *in vivo*. We discovered that experimental autoimmune encephalomyelitis (EAE), considered by many to be a model of MS, could be produced by clones of T cells reactive to myelin basic protein (MBP) (Ben-Nun and Cohen, 1982a). Intravenous administration of about 10^6 activated T cells specific for MBP led to EAE in naive recipient rats. This methodology made it possible to satisfy Koch's postulates and serially transfer EAE from rat to rat by re-isolating the original line of anti-MBP T cells (Naparstek et al., 1982). Activated anti-MBP T cells demonstrated the ability to migrate to the brain *in vivo* (Naparstek et al., 1983) and could damage central myelin in tissue culture (Yarom et al., 1983). Thus we were able to reduce EAE to specific anti-MPB T cells. Moreover, the cause of EAE could be reduced further to anti-MBP T cell receptors (TCRs), since it is mainly the TCR that distinguishes the different T cell clones (Cohen, 2000; Oksenberg et al., 1993b).

3. NECESSARY, BUT NOT SUFFICIENT

Soon after reducing EAE to pure cultures of anti-MBP T cells, my colleagues and I went on to transform the forbidden T cell clones into therapeutic reagents by a procedure called T cell vaccination. The idea was to use the autoimmune clones as a vaccine (Ben-Nun and Cohen, 1982a) to activate an anti-clonotypic (anti-idiotypic) response against the renegade cells (Elias et al., 1991) and so use the immune system itself to rid the body of the cause of EAE. T cell vaccination was found to be effective in EAE and in other experimental T cell mediated autoimmune diseases, and T cell vaccination is now being applied to the treatment of MS patients (Stinissen et al., 1998; Zhang et al., 1993). Thus there seems to be confirmatory evidence to support the idea that autoimmune T cells, with their autoimmune TCR, were the cause of autoimmune disease.

However, an idea may still be wrong despite the fact that the idea has produced a correct experiment. The flaw here is that autoimmune T cell clones may be necessary for disease, but they are not sufficient for disease. Rats which had recovered from EAE and were resistant to future bouts of the disease were found to harbor clones of potentially virulent anti-MBP T cells

(Ben-Nun and Cohen, 1982; Cohen, 1992; Mor and Cohen, 1993). Thus, EAE could not be reduced to the presence or absence of anti-MBP T cell clones; the clones were surely necessary but not sufficient for EAE. Thus, single aberrant clones of autoimmune lymphocytes are not the cause of autoimmune disease in the way that single aberrant clones of transformed cells are the cause of cancer. The insufficiency of anti-MBP T cells as the cause for EAE was reinforced by the findings that healthy rats are populated with anti-MBP T cells and, despite the presence of the clones, the rats will never develop EAE unless they are actively immunized to MBP or receive activated anti-MPB T cells (Ben-Nun and Cohen, 1982; Mor and Cohen, 1993). Anti-MBP T cells are also easily recovered from healthy people, and not only from persons with MS (Schluesener and Wekerle, 1985). In fact, anti-MBP T cells probably help maintain the central nervous system (CNS) in the face of trauma; we recently found that such cells mediate neuroprotection (Moalem et al., 1999). We did not know whether anti-MBP T cells are necessary for MS; the presence of such T cells is certainly not sufficient to cause MS. We must return to the question we raised above: can MS (or EAE) or other autoimmune diseases be reduced to a causal element that is both necessary and sufficient?

4. STRUCTURES

It is obvious that many structural elements are necessary to generate MS or EAE: MHC susceptibility genes, T cells with specific TCR types, target antigens and peptides presented in the nervous system, accessory molecules involved in T cell recognition and cell traffic, enzymes to penetrate tissues, inflammatory cytokines and inflammatory leukocytes, and so forth. But all of these elements are present in healthy persons. None of the elements is abnormal. What can there be wrong with healthy elements that allows them to cause a disease?

The search for the cause of MS has been frustrated because we tend to think of causality, in essence, as structural. We are satisfied intellectually when complex actions can be attributed to simple underlying structures (Cohen and Stewart, 1995). After all, structure determines function (Cohen, 2000). Water, for example, functions the way it does in biology as well as in chemistry because of the fundamental dipolar structure of the water molecule. An antibody recognizes its specific antigen by virtue of the structure of the antibody's combining site (Cohen, 2000). Many scientific explanations are founded, in principle, on the discovery of the basic structures responsible for the observed functions. In biology the reduction of function to defined structures is especially valuable because such discoveries, as stated at the outset, lead to rational therapy. All the complex expressions of sickle cell anemia can be understood to result from the structure of the gene for hemoglobin S. The diagnosis of a sick gene prescribes an ideal treatment, that of gene therapy, irrespective of whether gene therapy is presently feasible. Hepatitis is caused by the structure of a particular virus; thus the ideal therapy is to get rid of the virus (various options are conceivable). The principle of reduction to structure motivates rational therapeutic innovations in immunology, too.

The reduction of an autoimmune disease to the structure of the TCR is a diagnosis that entails particular therapies. If renegade clones are the culprits, then rational therapy would be to kill or inactivate the TCR-bearing T cells, or to block the recognition by the TCR of the MHC-target peptide complex. Interference with antigen recognition has been the aim of blocking peptides, antibodies to the MHC, to the MHC-peptide complex, to the TCR, or to other ancillary ligands involved in T cell recognition, such as the CD4 molecule (Bach, 1993). Is such structural reduction going to work in therapy for MS? Can we cure the disease by getting rid of some discrete structure?

5. INTERACTIONS

Despite the best efforts, I doubt whether we shall be able to cure MS by blocking or getting rid of some specific structure, either a cell or a molecule. This is because the disease MS is caused not by a T cell clone, a structure, but by an **interaction**, the way the T cell clone interacts with other lymphocytes, with the blood vessels and the CNS. The disease is caused by the fact that the clones are activated in the CNS in a way that leads them to secrete pro-inflammatory cytokines, IFN-γ, TNF-α and others, which generate damaging inflammation leading to demyelination and the signs and symptoms of MS (Panitch et al., 1987; Sharief and Hentges, 1991). Thus, MS and EAE cannot be reduced to discrete structures, but to interactions between structures, undesirable interactions between otherwise healthy structures (Cohen, 2000).

For clarity, reduction to interactions might need a terminology to distinguish this type of causality from reduction to structure. The term **interactional causality** might be suitable because the effect emerges from a context of interactions rather than from a specific underlying structure.

6. INTERACTIONAL THERAPY

If autoimmune diseases are caused by interactions and not by underlying structures, should we change the way we do basic and clinical research in the autoimmune field? The answer depends on how one looks at the question. As in the past, we still must persist in the classical work of structural, reductive science and identify the various cells and molecules that are necessary to produce MS (Cohen, 2000). But we would probably do better to think about the disease process more comprehensively and consider the context of interactions of these cells and molecules. In other words, autoimmune diseases will have to be reduced to their requisite structural ingredients: genes, gene products and other molecules and cells. But we probably would not be able to cure the disease rationally (we might stumble onto the cure by accident) unless we consider the critical interactions. The cure will come not by **inactivating** any of the key structural elements, but rather by using key structural elements to **activate** new or corrective interactions (Cohen, 1995).

A concrete example of therapeutic activation has emerged from the work of my colleagues and me on the spontaneous autoimmune diabetes developing in non-obese diabetic NOD strain mice. We began by identifying some key structural elements that were not previously thought to be involved in the disease. We discovered that T cells reactive to a stress protein, the 60 kDa heat shock protein (hsp60) of the mouse, could mediate disease in healthy recipient mice (Elias et al., 1990; 1994). The anti-hsp60 T cells were not sufficient to cause diabetes because healthy individuals also harbor such T cells (Munk et al., 1989). Nevertheless, the pathogenic T cells served as a probe to help us identify a target peptide in the hsp60 molecule (Elias and Cohen, 1994; Elias et al., 1991). We then went on to test the interactions of the hsp60 peptide and how it could influence the autoimmune diabetic process. The peptide was found to activate opposing effects depending on the context of its administration. Conjugated to a foreign carrier molecule, the self-peptide could activate an autoimmune effector response leading to insulitis and hyperglycemia (Elias et al., 1995). In contrast, the same peptide unconjugated to another immunogen could induce the arrest of the autoimmune process, even when it was far advanced (Elias and Cohen, 1994; Elias and Cohen, 1995). It is now clear that hsp60 – peptide therapy activates a burst of peptide-specific Th2-type T cells (producing anti-inflammatory cytokines IL-4, IL-10 and probably TGF-β) that abort the inflammatory process produced by the Th1-type T cells (producing IFN-γ and IL-2) that actually penetrate the islets and inactivate the insulin-producing β cells (Elias et al., 1997). The Th2-type of interaction resets the cytokine profile and down-regulates the Th1-type responses to other β-cell antigens such as insulin and glutamic acid decarboxylase. Interestingly, therapeutic vaccination with the hsp60 target peptide led to the activation of anti-idiotypic T cells that recognized the T cell receptor of the pathogenic autoimmune T cells (Elias et al., 1999). In other words, the Th2 cytokine shift was accompanied by anti-idiotypic regulation; both forms of immune regulation would seem to be linked functionally. Most importantly, these modifications of the autoimmune interaction are expressed clinically as to cure advanced disease in the majority of the mice (Elias and Cohen, 1995). Therapeutic peptide vaccination is now being tested clinically in humans suffering from recent onset type 1 diabetes mellitus.

In this example, we see that the cells and molecules that structure the immune system can be left intact and that only their interactions need be influenced by a key control element to shift the system away from a pathogenic interaction (Cohen, 2000).

7. THERAPY FOR MS

I would now like to discuss the prospects for specific immune modulation of a disease such as MS. If we perceive MS to be caused by pathogenic interactions, then it makes sense to try and activate the immune system using information that will induce corrective or new interactions within the autoimmune response that causes MS (Cohen, 1995). In other words, MS might be susceptible not to immune suppression, but to immune activation. T cell-vaccination (Ben-Nun et al., 1981b) is one way of activating immune regulation (Elias et al., 1991; Lider et al., 1988) and clinical trials are underway (Stinissen et al., 1998; Zhang et al., 1993). Of course, we can also consider exploiting the Th1-Th2 paradigm; epitopes of MBP or other relevant antigens might be administered in a cytokine or adjuvant context that activates a switch from a pro-inflammatory outcome to an anti-inflammatory outcome of the autoimmune response (Ablamunits et al., 1998; Elias et al., 1997). The success of the activation approach, using either T cell or peptide vaccinations, would depend on two conditions: the activation would have to be given early in the course of disease, or during the early remitting phase. Once MS progresses to a chronic unremitting phase, the disease process has become robustly entrenched and may no longer be susceptible to interactive manipulation. Indeed, the capacity of MS to remit spontaneously can be taken as evidence that the autoimmune response is still naturally susceptible to shifting interactions.

A second condition for activation therapy is that we discover surrogate markers for the pathogenic and for the therapeutic types of interaction. We need surrogate markers because we cannot wait for years to pass to see the outcome of therapy. We must know if we are on the right track. Has the patient responded as we desire? Is the dose of peptide sufficient for the particular patient? Is a booster activation needed? If, for example, secretion of IFN-γ by anti-MBP T cells were a sign of a pathogenic interaction and secretion of IL-4, IL-10 or TGF-β were signs of a healthy interaction, then we could use such markers to tailor activation therapy to the patient's needs. Time will tell.

Acknowledgment. I am the incumbent of the Mauerberger Chair of Immunology, the Director of the Robert Koch-Minerva Center for Research in Autoimmune Diseases. I thank Ms. Danielle Sabah-Israel for her help in preparing this manuscript.

REFERENCES

Ablamunits V., Elias D., Reshef T. and Cohen I. R. (1998): Islet T cells secreting IFN-gamma in NOD mouse diabetes: arrest by p277 peptide treatment. J. Autoimmun., **11**, 73–81.

Bach J. F. (1993): Immunosuppressive therapy of autoimmune diseases. Immunol. Today, **14**, 322–326.

Ben-Nun A. and Cohen I. R. (1982): Spontaneous remission and acquired resistance to autoimmune encephalomyelitis (EAE) are associated with suppression of T cell reactivity: suppressed EAE effector T cells recovered as T cell lines. J. Immunol., **128**, 1450–1457.

Ben-Nun A., Wekerle H. and Cohen I. R. (1981a): The rapid isolation of clonable antigen-specific T lymphocyte lines capable of mediating autoimmune encephalomyelitis. Eur. J. Immunol., **11**, 195–199.

Ben-Nun A., Wekerle H. and Cohen I. R. (1981b): Vaccination against autoimmune encephalomyelitis with T lymphocyte line cells reactive against myelin basic protein. Nature, **292**, 60–61.

Bronze M. S. and Dale J. B. (1996): The reemergence of serious group A streptococcal infections and acute rheumatic fever. Am. J. Med. Sci., **311**, 411–454.

Burnet F. M. (1969): Self and not-self. University Press, Cambridge.

Cohen I. R. (1992): The cognitive paradigm and the immunological homunculus. Immunol. Today, **13**, 490–494.

Cohen I. R. (1995): Treatment of autoimmune disease: to activate or to deactivate? Chem. Immunol., **60**, 150–160.

Cohen I. R. (2000): Tending Adam's garden. Evolving the cognitive immune self. Academic Press, London, UK.

Cohen J. and Stewart I. (1995): The collapse of chaos. Discovering simplicity in a complex world. Penguin Books, New York.

Ebers G. C., Bulman D. E., Sadovnick A. D., Paty D. W., Warren S., Hader W., Murray T. J., Seland T. P., Duquette P., Grey T., Nelson R., Nicolle M. and Brunet D. (1986): A population based study of multiple sclerosis in twins. N. Engl. J. Med., **315**, 1638–1642.

Elias D. and Cohen I. R. (1994): Peptide therapy for diabetes in NOD mice. Lancet, **343**, 704–706.

Elias D. and Cohen I. R. (1995): Treatment of autoimmune diabetes in NOD mice. Diabetes, **44**, 1132–1138.

Elias D., Marcus H., Reshef T., Ablumunits V. and Cohen I. R. (1995): Induction of diabetes in standard mice by immunization to the p277 peptide of a 60 kDa heat shock protein. Eur. J. Immunol., **25**, 2851–2857.

Elias D., Markovits D., Reshef T., van der Zee R. and Cohen I. R. (1990): Induction and therapy of autoimmune diabetes in the non-obese diabetic (NOD/Lt) mouse by a 65-kDa heat shock protein. Proc. Natl. Acad. Sci. USA, **87**, 1576–1580.

Elias D., Meilin A., Ablamunits V., Birk O. S., Carmi P., Konen-Waisman S. and Cohen I. R. (1997): Hsp60 peptide therapy of NOD mouse diabetes induces a TH2 cytokine burst and downregulates autoimmunity to various beta-cells antigens. Diabetes, **46**, 758–764.

Elias D., Prigozin H., Polak N., Rapoport M., Lohse A. W. and Cohen I. R. (1994): Autoimmune diabetes induced by the beta-cell toxin STZ. Immunity to the 60-kDa heat shock protein and to insulin. Diabetes, **43**, 992–998.

Elias D., Reshef T., Birk O. S., van der Zee R., Walker M. D. and Cohen I. R. (1991): Vaccination against autoimmune mouse diabetes with a T-cell epitope of the human 65-kDa heat shock protein. Proc. Natl. Acad. Sci. USA, **88**, 3088–3091.

Elias D., Tikochinsky Y., Frankel G. and Cohen I. R. (1999): Regulation of NOD mouse autoimmune diabetes by T cells that recognize a T-cell receptor CDR3 peptide. Int. Immunol., **11**, 957–966.

Gill F. M., Sleeper L. A., Wiener S. J., Brown A. K., Bellevue R., Grover R., Pegelow C. H. and Vichinsky E. (1995): Clinical events in the first decade in a cohort of infants with sickle cell disease. Blood, **86**, 776–783.

Lider O., Reshef T., Beraud E., Ben-Nun A. and Cohen I. R. (1988): Anti-idiotypic network induced by T cell vaccination against experimental autoimmune encephalomyelitis. Science, **239**, 181–183.

Moalem G., Leibowitz-Amit R., Yoles E., Mor F., Cohen I. R. and Schwartz M. (1999): Autoimmune T cells protect neurons from secondary degeneration after central nervous system axotomy. Nat. Med., **5**, 49–55.

Mor F. and Cohen I. R. (1993): Shifts in the epitopes of myelin basic protein recognized by Lewis rat T cells before, during and after the induction of experimental autoimmune encephalomyelitis. J. Clin. Invest., **92**, 2199–2206.

Munk E. M., Schoel B., Modrow S., Karr R. W., Young R. A. and Kaufmann S. H. E. (1989): T lymphocytes from healthy individuals with specificity to self-epitopes shared by the mycobacteria and human 65-kilodalton heat shock protein. J. Immunol., **143**, 2844–2849.

Naparstek Y., Ben-Nun A., Holoshitz J., Reshef T., Frenkel A., Rosenberg M. and Cohen I. R. (1983): T lymphocyte lines producing or vaccinating against autoimmune encephalomyelitis (EAE): functional activation induces PNA receptors and accumulation in the brain and thymus of line cells. Eur. J. Immunol., **13**, 418–423.

Naparstek Y., Holoshitz J., Eisenstein S., Reshef T., Rappaport S., Chemke J., Ben-Nun A. and

Cohen I. R. (1982): Effector T lymphocyte line cells migrate to the thymus and persist there. Nature, **300**, 262–263.

Oksenberg J. R., Begovich A. B., Erlich H. A. and Steinman L. (1993a): Genetic factors in MS. JAMA, **270**, 2352–2359.

Oksenberg J. R., Panzara M. A., Begovich A. B., Mitchell D., Erlich H. A., Murray R. S., Shimonkevitz R., Sherritt M., Rothbard J., Bernard C. C. and Steinman L. (1993b): Selection for T cell receptor Vβ-Dβ-Jβ gene rearrangements with specificity for a myelin basic protein peptide in brain lesions of multiple sclerosis. Nature, **362**, 68–70.

Panitch H. S., Hirsch R. L., Schindler J. and Johnson K. P. (1987): Treatment of multiple sclerosis with gamma interferon: exacerbations associated with activation of the immune system. Neurology, **37**, 1097–1102.

Schluesener H. J. and Wekerle H. (1985): Autoaggressive T lymphocyte lines recognizing the encephalitogenic region of myelin basic protein: *in vitro* selection from unprimed rat T lymphocyte populations. J. Immunol., **135**, 3128–3133.

Sharief M. K. and Hentges R. (1991): Association between TNF-α and disease progression in patients with MS. N. Engl. J. Med., **325**, 467–472.

Stinissen P., Medaer R. and Raus J. (1998): Preliminary data of an extended open label phase 1 study of T cell vaccination in multiple sclerosis (abstract). J. Neuroimmunol., **90**, 99.

Vyse T. J. and Todd J. A. (1996): Genetic analysis of autoimmune disease. Cell, **85**, 311–313.

Yarom Y., Lev-Ram V., Naparstek Y., Holoshitz J., Ben-Nun A. and Cohen I. R. (1983): Immunospecific inhibition of nerve conduction by T lymphocytes reactive to basic protein of myelin. Nature, **303**, 246–247.

Zhang J., Medaer R., Stinissen P., Hafler D. and Raus J. (1993): MHC-restricted depletion of human basic protein-reactive T cells by T cell vaccination. Science, **261**, 1451–1454.

UNCOVERING THE DIFFERENCES BETWEEN T CELL TOLERANCE AND IMMUNITY

ANTHONY T. VELLA

Department of Microbiology, Oregon State University, Corvallis, Oregon, USA

Abstract In the last two decades, T cell function has been analyzed *in vitro* from many different angles, with a great deal of attention dedicated to the basic requirements of activation. During this time, a compendium of information has been collected and has proven to be invaluable. Paradoxically, very little is known about T cell activation and function *in vivo*. In the last decade, a number of models have been developed which allow the tracking of Ag-activated T cells *in vivo* and these studies have been instrumental in advancing the field of T cell biology. In particular, a new and emerging paradigm of T cell immunity is evolving.

Key words: T cell activation; immunity; immune memory.

1. DEFINING ACTIVATION, TOLERANCE AND MEMORY

The larger part of this review is dedicated to examining CD4 T cell tolerance versus CD4 T cell activation. Activation is a somewhat confusing word as we do not define activation in the same way for each circumstance. For example, one who studies signal transduction may define activation by the ligation of a receptor, while a molecular biologist may consider the induction of gene expression as activation. Further, a cell biologist may regard proliferation or protein secretion as another form of activation. Depending on the subdiscipline of immunology being discussed, all of these definitions of activation may be applicable. Nevertheless, in the context of immunobiology, none of them may be accurate. Therefore, for the sake of clarity, I will deal with this issue by using the term "immunity", which translates to development of memory.

It seems that defining memory is much easier than defining tolerance. Memory is the ability of the immune system to recall a response against an antigen (Ag). In simple terms, being immune is equated with memory resulting from a previous exposure to an Ag. For example, one is immune to a pre-

A. Górski et al. (eds.), Autoimmunity, 11–26.

viously injected Ag but is not usually able to mount an anamnestic response to an Ag to which the subject has never been exposed. Normally, a memory response is more vigorous than the initial response. The complexity of this issue is confounded when one begins to ask whether there are varying degrees of memory and why all memory responses are not equivalent. For example, why are certain vaccine strategies more effective than others? This latter point may be related to tolerance induction.

T cell tolerance to Ag is believed to occur in at least two sites in the body: the thymus (central tolerance) and the periphery (peripheral tolerance) (Marrack et al., 1993; Sprent et al., 1988). One other site is in the gut (Weiner, 1997). Tolerance in the thymus occurs during T cell development. As T cells differentiate into mature cells, they are screened for their ability to bind to peptides presented by major histocompatibility complex (MHC) molecules. The details of this process are not the focal point of this review and, therefore, I will only touch on the subject. Briefly, as T cells become double positive ($CD4^+$ $CD8^+$) expressing cells, they begin to survey MHC/peptide complexes and, if the affinity of the T cell receptor (TCR) for its ligand reaches beyond a certain threshold, the cell will then be programmed to die via apoptosis (Anderson et al., 1999). Negative selection also takes place in the bone marrow to eliminate self-reactive B cells.

Peripheral tolerance appears to be a more complicated process. Affinity of the TCR for MHC/pcptide may play a role, but costimulatory molecules are also intimately involved, thereby complicating the situation even further. Similarly, understanding the end result of tolerance induction becomes a challenge because the readout of tolerance is hard to quantify. In the case of memory it is very clear what one looks for, namely, a recall response that can be measured by cell proliferation, cytokine production or target cell lysis. In the case of tolerance there should be little response to measure since the T cell is tolerant to the Ag. This raises several important issues: are T cells present but unresponsive (i.e. anergy), have they migrated to other parts of the body and, therefore, are unable to interact with the Ag, or are they dead? It may be that tolerance is a result of all of these processes to varying degrees. For example, it makes sense that a cell which is on its way to death will have little ability to produce cytokines or proliferate. In this case the cell would appear anergic but is simply moribund.

2. MODELS OF T CELL TOLERANCE

There are several models of T cell tolerance that have allowed investigators to distinguish between these possibilities. The one commonality between each of these models is the ability to track Ag-activated T cells. This is critical, because it allows one to determine whether the cell population in question is present or not. Initial studies came from the use of superAg's (SAg) (Marrack and Kappler, 1990). Early on it was noticed that T cells would be eliminated in the thymus of mouse strains which expressed mls proteins reactive to those T cells (Morrissey et al., 1983). Later, soluble bacterial SAg was used to induce tolerance in mice. This later model has led to a number of important discoveries. For example, the use of SAg facilitated the discovery of T cell negative selection in the thymus (Kappler et al., 1987). Additionally, in the periphery it was found that SAg activation induced T cell death through an apoptotic mechanism (Kawabe and Ochi, 1991). SAg's have also been implicated in a vast number of human afflictions (Bernal et al., 1999; Kotzin et al., 1993). Two of the foremost examples are food poisoning and toxic shock syndrome.

The SAg model is invaluable as a system to study peripheral tolerance. The key feature of the system is the ability to follow SAg-activated T cells over time based on the TCR Vβ chain that they bear. Therefore, monoclonal antibodies (mAb) specific to TCR Vβ chains can be used to follow activated T cells directly *ex vivo* through the use of a flow cytometer. It is widely known that as T cells are stimulated by SAg they will respond by blasting, producing cytokines and proliferating. Moreover, *in vivo* data has shown that SAg-specific T cells (both CD4- and CD8-bearing) will respond to SAg by clonally expanding, such that the numbers of SAg-reactive T cells are significantly higher than in uninjected mice (Marrack and Kappler, 1990). Expansion peaks by 2 to 3 days after SAg injection and is followed by mass deletion of the responding cells. Deletion is usually completed by one week after injection and the vast majority of these cells die by apoptosis (Kawabe and Ochi, 1991). Notwithstanding, it has been shown that these cells can also become anergic (Cauley et al., 1997; Kawabe and Ochi et al., 1990).

A second model developed by the Jenkins laboratory utilizes transgenic TCR-expressing T cells (Kearney et al., 1994). These cells are adoptively transferred into genetically similar wild-type mice such that the proportion of CD4 TCR transgenic T cells is approximately 1%. This low percentage of Ag-reactive T cells mimics physiological conditions and allows the T cells to be tracked after responding to the Ag. After T cell transfer, the mouse is injected with Ag and the T cells can then be monitored using an anti-idiotypic TCR mAb. The results of the SAg model and this model are generally very similar. Models which utilize transgenic TCR CD8 T cells specific to viral peptides have also been very useful (Zinkernagel et al., 1999).

Before the use of these models, it was impossible to determine the fate of the Ag-responsive cells *in vivo*. Earlier systems compared the physical state of the Ag more than the fate of T and B cell functions. In a set of pinnacle studies in the early 1960's by Dresser (Dresser, 1962; Dresser and Gowland, 1964), it was shown that small amounts of bovine γ globulin were tolerogenic in mice compared to larger doses. At the same time, Dresser noted that high--speed spins, which removed aggregated proteins, were essential for tolerogenicity. Even earlier studies by Freund (1951) showed the positive effects of various adjuvant oils on antibody synthesis. Paradoxically, it is still not clear how adjuvants specifically function to boost immunity. Taken together, the physical state of the Ag and the form of presentation can determine the quantity and quality of a lymphocyte response.

3. HOW COSTIMULATORY SIGNALS AFFECT T CELL TOLERANCE AND IMMUNITY

Differential signaling for tolerance induction over immunity was first proposed by Bretscher and Cohn in 1970. Specifically, they proposed that binding of one determinant by a surface antibody receptor alone would lead to tolerance, but this signal in conjunction with a carrier antibody molecule binding a second determinant would lead to antibody induction. Later, Lafferty and Cunningham (1975) modified this idea. They proposed that two signals were needed to drive alloreactions. Signal one, Ag recognition (this is the same as the Bretscher and Cohn model) and signal two, or the costimulatory signal, are derived from the antigen-presenting cell (APC). Some years later this model was confirmed with a series of *in vivo* and *in vitro* experiments performed by the Schwartz laboratory (see below).

Chemical modification of APC by treatment with the crosslinker 1-ethyl--3-(3-dimethylaminopropyl)-carbodiimide was shown to induce Ag-specific unresponsiveness in mice (Jenkins and Schwartz, 1987). The results suggested that signal one without signal two induced tolerance in the Ag-activated lymphocyte population. Modified APC, in contrast to unmanipulated APC, were able to deliver signal 1 but were unable to deliver signal 2. A few years later a mAb was produced against murine CD28 and definitive evidence for a second signal was established (Harding et al., 1992). CD28 is expressed on T cells at all times and is expressed on immature T cells in the thymus (Gross et al., 1992). The ligand for CD28 is B7-1 (CD80) and B7-2 (CD86), which are expressed on APC (Harris and Ronchese, 1999). In general, dendritic cells constitutively express these B7 molecules, but all other APC need to become activated in order for B7 expression to occur.

In the presence of signal 1 and signal 2, naïve T cells will increase stability of IL-2 mRNA, synthesize IL-2, increase expression of the IL-2R and then begin to clonally expand (Jenkins et al., 1987b; Powell et al., 1998). This is the essence of the two-signal hypothesis. Effector T cells, on the other hand, do not seem to be as dependent on CD28 costimulation (Croft and Dubey, 1997). They are capable of secreting large quantities of cytokines without costimulation. Memory T cells also seem to be dependent on costimulation, but perhaps to a lesser degree than to naïve T cells (Dutton et al., 1998). Thus, during the differentiation of T cells after signals 1 and 2 multiple signaling pathways must be rewired to allow effector cell activation without costimulation. Currently it is not clear whether CD4 T cell effectors develop into memory cells or whether memory cells develop from a totally different cell lineage.

When naïve T cells are stimulated in the presence of signal 1 but in the absence of signal 2, these cells will become anergic. Anergy means the T cells do not proliferate and fail to make IL-2. Anergic T cell clones, however, produce other cytokines such as IFN-γ and IL-3 when stimulated (Jenkins et al., 1987a). In general, Th2 cells can also be induced to become anergic (Yssel et al., 1994). In doing so they will fail to provide help to B cells and be unable to proliferate. Thus, the two-signal model has allowed immunologists to compartmentalize T cell responses in a logical and manageable fashion.

Several confusing issues remain with regard to the two-signal hypothesis. In theory, constitutive B7 expression on circulating or localized APC should dramatically increase the likelihood of autoimmunity. In an elegant set of *in vivo* experiments, it was shown that constitutive B7 expression within the pancreas did not induce diabetes unless these transgenic mice were crossed with TNF-α transgenic mice which secrete (Guerder et al., 1994). Thus, signal one (self-pancreatic peptides) and signal two (transgenic CD80) were not sufficient to stimulate autoimmunity and, therefore, the two-signal model may be an oversimplification for long-lasting T cell activation *in vivo*. In a related set of experiments, it was shown that $CD28^{-/-}$ mice can clear certain viral infections and are able to generate protective responses to parasites even though these mice are less capable of generating memory T cells (Shahinian et al., 1993; Villegas et al., 1999). These data suggest several important hypotheses and notions: 1) since two signals are not enough to stimulate autoimmunity, it is likely that other signals are important; 2) there must be other costimulatory signals which are sufficient to function in the absence of CD28 and the question is whether they function when CD28 is present. Taken together, we can conclude that two signals are sufficient to "activate" naïve T cells *in vitro* and *in vivo*, but T cell immunity *in vivo* is likely to involve multiple signals. Additionally, the difference between autoimmunity and tolerance induction is more complicated than competition for signal 2 and likely involves the action of proinflammatory cytokines such as TNF-α.

CD40 is a member of the TNF/NGF superfamily of receptors. CD40 is expressed on all APC, amongst other cell types, and its ligand CD154 (formally known as gp39 or CD40-ligand) is expressed on activated T cells (Grewal and Flavell, 1996). CD154 binding to surface CD40 on APC enhances expression of CD80 and CD86 (Kiener et al., 1995; Roy et al., 1995). In turn, these APC are able to provide T cells with costimulation. Specifically, B cell surface Ig binding to its specific target (B cell signal 1) is not sufficient to induce expression of costimulatory molecules and, therefore, will induce anergy unless given signal 2. CD154 bearing T cells can interact with resting B cells, which express a peptide/MHC complex that the T cell can recognize. CD154 will bind to CD40 (B cell signal 2), thereby causing up-regulation of CD80 and CD86. This will promote B cell activation and further T cell activation. How does the original T cell become activated so that it expresses CD154? Most likely this is through an activated macrophage or dendritic cell, which are probably activated nonspecifically by pathogens or adjuvants.

Although the CD40/CD154 system explains how T and B cells can communicate with each other, several important questions remain: How much time is required for this interaction? How many hits between T and B cells are necessary for full activation? Can the degree of interaction lead to different functional outcomes for T and B cells? The answers to these questions and others will provide important clues towards our understanding of immunity.

Other members of the TNF/NGF superfamily of receptors are also very important during immunity. OX40 is a receptor that is expressed on Ag-stimulated T cells that shows structural homology to CD40 (Weinberg et al., 1998). *In vivo* experiments have indicated that OX40 is expressed predominantly on CD4 T cells and not significantly on CD8 T cells (Paterson et al., 1987). OX40-ligand is restricted in its expression, but is found on activated APC (Stuber et al., 1995). OX40-ligand stimulation on B cells induces differentiation and contributes to Ig synthesis. Also, stimulation of OX40-ligand on dendritic cells leads to enhanced secretion of proinflammatory cytokines (Ohshima et al., 1997). Collectively, these results suggest that OX40/OX40--ligand stimulation will improve immune responses *in vivo*.

Several key features concerning OX40 are now well established. OX40 stimulation on activated T cells leads to enhanced proliferation (Paterson et al., 1987). This result is also evident when Th1 and Th2 cells are examined, showing that there is no bias toward one population over the other (Weinberg et al., 1998). This is supportive of *in vivo* data showing that OX40 stimulation can promote Th2 responses (Flynn et al., 1998). Additionally, it has been shown that OX40 and CD28 engagement on naïve T cells synergistically promote proliferation and IL-2 production (Gramaglia et al., 1998). Therefore,

OX40 operates in a similar fashion to CD28 as a potent costimulatory signal for T cells.

4-1BB is another member of this family that shares a few structural and functional similarities to the other members (Vinay and Kwon, 1998). In contrast to OX40, 4-1BB has been characterized as an activation molecule that is expressed on CD4 and CD8 T cells (Pollok et al., 1993). 4-1BB stimulation in mice carrying tumors leads to enhanced tumor regression (Melero et al., 1997). In these mice, CD8 T cells possessed higher cytotoxic T lymphocyte (CTL) activity and exhibited a more robust cytokine response (Shuford et al., 1997).

In our studies we found that 4-1BB was indeed expressed on both CD4 and CD8 staphylococcal enterotoxin A (SEA)-activated T cells, but the CD8 T cells expressed more of this molecule and enhanced 4-1BB expression was seen much earlier after Ag-stimulation (Takahashi et al., 1999). When mice were injected with both SEA and an agonist mAb specific to 4-1BB, we found that proliferation was enhanced in the presence of the mAb. This is similar to what is observed by stimulating OX40 or CD28 on SEA-activated T cells *in vivo*. In contrast, however, 4-1BB stimulation led to a significant block in peripheral deletion, whereas the other two did not. Oddly enough, we found that the CD8 T cells were protected from deletion, but the CD4 T cells were still deleted. One possibility to explain this data is that 4-1BB is wired differently on CD8 versus CD4 T cells. Future experiments on the subject of comparing 4-1BB signaling between CD4 and CD8 T cells should be very interesting.

4. THE INFLUENCE OF CYTOKINES ON T CELL SURVIVAL AND MEMORY

The existence of T cell memory has been recognized for a number of years (Dutton et al., 1998). For much of this time there has been an ongoing debate concerning the importance of Ag in maintaining memory. For the most part this debate continues, but for CD8 T cells there seems to be little doubt that Ag is not essential (Hou et al., 1994; Lau et al., 1994; Mullbacher, 1994). For CD4 T cells it is still unclear as to the role of Ag, however, earlier reports show that memory T cells can survive in the absence of Ag (Gray and Matzinger, 1991). Nevertheless, this contradicts previous studies, and so the debate continues (Swain, 1994).

The process of memory T cell generation is not well understood and represents one of the last great frontiers in basic immunology. Part of the reason this has been difficult to study is the lack of understanding of what constitutes memory. This has generated a wide spectrum of viewpoints and raises a variety of immunological questions, including: 1) are memory cells derived from effectors, 2) how many signals do T cells require to become memory cells, 3) how different are memory T cells from naïve cells, 4) where are memory cells located in the body and 5) how do memory cells avoid death signals? For the past decade only a few tenets have been established with regard to these and other questions (Dutton et al., 1998). First, memory cells are usually CD44hi, CD62-l negative and CD45RO positive. Secondly, memory T cells do seem to respond more vigorously to stimuli than naïve T cells. And thirdly, recent data have shown that memory CD8 T cells are derived from effector cells and are not a separate lineage (Opferman, 1999). Although there may be examples when these tenets do not hold, in general they should be viewed as guidelines.

One of the more pressing issues is how effector cells are instructed to become memory cells. Recently, it has been shown that at least five cellular divisions are necessary for effector CTLs to develop into memory cells (Opferman, 1999). These data raise the question of what occurs during these divisions? Secondly, are these cells qualitatively different from the cells which have undergone <5 divisions, or have these cells out-competed the other cells for growth factors? These questions raise the issue of whether a subpopulation of effector cells possesses a selective advantage in obtaining a memory phenotype. For example, as T cells begin to clonally expand, it may be possible that a small proportion of effector cells receives a limiting signal(s) which grooms these cells to divide further and differentiate into memory cells. Potential signals which may drive this process are cytokines, accessory molecules on neighboring cells as they divide, or perhaps the lack of a death signal. Regardless of the outcome, these studies will lead to new and exciting concepts in immunology.

Another aspect of memory acquisition is the necessity of T cells to survive through the effector phase. It is widely believed that, as T cells progress to effector cells, a number of cell death mechanisms are activated. These include receptor-mediated death pathways such as Fas and trail, cytokine deprivation, and, possibly, steroid-induced death (Krammer et al., 1994). Regardless of the mechanism, effector T cells must thwart this attack in order to survive. Therefore, T cells have developed ways in which death can be circumvented.

Earlier it was noted by Chiller and Weigle (1973) that tolerance could be circumvented by administration of adjuvant. Specifically, they demonstrated that lipopolysaccharide (LPS) and soluble IgG induced immunity whereas soluble IgG alone induced tolerance. Some years later this study was expanded upon, using a SAg model which utilized SEA as the SAg (Vella et al.,

1995). Injection of SEA leads to profound deletion of the TCR Vβ3-reactive T cells (McCormack et al., 1993). If LPS is injected at the time of or one day after SEA injection, deletion is significantly inhibited. This was true for CD4 and CD8 T cells. Upon further examination, these rescued cells were found to be responsive to SEA and, therefore, were not anergic (Vella et al., 1996). Mechanistically, it was shown that TNF-α was the critical factor in mediating rescue, since TNF-α neutralizing mAb inhibited LPS-induced rescue (Vella et al., 1995). In an analogous experiment, injection of TNF-α and SEA led to rescue from deletion (Vella et al., 1997b). LPS seems to fit the description of a "danger" signal as proposed by Matzinger (1994; 1998).

The irony of these results is that TNF-α is a well-noted death-inducing cytokine (Zheng et al., 1995). In a related scenario, it has been known for some time that the quintessential death receptor, Fas (CD95), can also be mitogenic when ligated (Alderson et al., 1993). Therefore, many factors must contribute to these types of differential responses, with microenvironment being no less important than any other. For example, cytokines may play a role in skewing one response over the other. This could be imagined in at least two ways. First, the quantity of certain cytokines in the microenvironment may promote survival over death. Large amounts of growth factors may block T cell apoptosis, whereas small amounts may not. A case in point is IL-2, which in large quantities will promote growth, but in small quantities will induce death via growth factor withdrawal (Kuroda et al., 1996; Lenardo, 1991). A second example suggests that the balance of various cytokines may influence survival over death. Exposure of activated T cells to proinflammatory cytokines may lead to one type of response, whereas anti-inflammatory cytokines may promote another. Additionally, there are certain cytokines, such as TGF-β, which have been characterized as having pleiotropic effects on cells, and TNF-α is no exception to this class of cytokines (Wahl, 1994). Thus, receptor activation driving a response in one circumstance and not in another is compatible with the idea that the outcome of an immune response is dependent upon multiple factors.

The mechanism of how TNF-α promotes T cell survival *in vivo* is unknown. Initial attempts were focused on analyzing a role for CD28 and B7. It was found that rescue was observed in mice treated with SEA/LPS and CTLA4-Ig as well as in CD28$^{-/-}$ mice (Vella et al., 1997a). These data strongly suggested that long-term survival was not driven by CD28 ligation. To investigate what role CD28 did play during SEA-induced proliferation, mice were given SEA and CTLA4-Ig and the fate of Vβ3 T cells was tracked. It was shown that the responsive cells did not grow to the same extent and deleted faster when CD28 ligation was blocked. One possibility to explain these data is that CD28 was not ligated efficiently. Therefore, experiments were conducted in which CD28 would be ligated maximally by activated APC *in vivo*. Injection of anti-CD40 led to dramatic increases of surface B7 expression (Kiener et al., 1995; Roy et al., 1995). SEA and anti-CD40 led to massive increases in clonal expansion, but deletion was not inhibited (Maxwell et al., 1999). Blocking CD28 from ligation in this model completely inhibited CD4 T cell clonal growth. Therefore, these data collectively show that signal 2 is a growth signal, but not a long-term survival signal *in vivo*.

These data led to the hypothesis that three signals may provide optimal *in vivo* immunity (Maxwel et al., 2000), these being Ag, costimulation and a survival signal. This notion is currently being tested and initial results are supportive of this idea. Nevertheless, one must remember that 4-1BB ligation induced clonal expansion and selective rescue of the CD8, but not CD4 T cells (Takahashi et al., 1999). In this case only two signals were necessary; however, it is unknown whether more costimulation or survival stimuli would enhance rescue.

Identifying survival signals has been actively pursued by a number of laboratories in a variety of systems. Recent reports have shown that IL-6 is a potent inhibitor of the spontaneously induced death of naïve T cells (Teague et al., 1997). Additionally, two members of the IL-2 family of cytokines, IL-4 and IL-7, can also block spontaneous death (Vella et al., 1997b). When T cells are activated and set up for death by growth factor withdrawal, IL-2, -4, -7 and -15 can all block death (Akbar et al., 1996; Vella et al., 1998). Interestingly, IL-2 and IL-15 induce survival with proliferation and IL-4 and IL-7 induce survival without proliferation. This is especially true with resting T cells, where rescue from apoptosis by IL-4, -6 and -7 was not associated with proliferation. This is even more intriguing when one considers the fact that IL-2, -4, -7 and -15 utilize a common receptor sub-unit for signaling (Leonard et al., 1994). Therefore, survival can occur via proliferation and in the absence of proliferation. Taken together, survival signals come in at least two varieties: ones that promote proliferation and others that do not. The mechanism which promotes one mode of action over the other will clearly involve the untangling of various signaling pathways and gene activation.

5. CLOSING THOUGHTS

Understanding the differences that drive tolerance versus immunity go beyond an academic exercise. These data are invaluable in our pursuit for an understanding of autoimmune disease, tumor immunology, infectious disease and vaccine development. Developing techniques that inhibit T cell growth will most certainly play a role in controlling autoimmune disease. Conversely, assisting T cell growth and survival will improve vaccine development by converting weak vaccines into potent ones. The greatest challenge, however, will be to control Ag-specific T cell function and avoid affecting cells that are bystanders. For example, it would be very dangerous to enhance global T cell growth for vaccination purposes in a patient who is suffering from an autoimmune disease. There will be a necessity to target the appropriate cells while sparing potentially dangerous cells.

A key characteristic of vaccination and in the establishment of autoimmune disease is the association of inflammatory responses. In almost all circumstances of autoimmune disease there seems to be a chronic inflammatory reaction. At the same time many of these autoimmune diseases, including arthritis and multiple sclerosis, are indeed dependent on T cells (Taneja and David, 1999). It is likely that this relationship between inflammation and pathogenic T cell responses is not a coincidence. Based on the data reviewed here, it is likely that proinflammatory cytokines are playing a role in keeping T cells alive. In particular, TNF-α is directly associated with this phenomenon. Additionally, a number of pathogenic organisms are associated with certain autoimmune diseases (Hausmann and Wucherpfennig, 1997). It could be predicted that these organisms provide the ammunition to induce an inflammatory response, which in turn potently activates T cells and that some of these T cells may be autoreactive. In the context of an appropriate inflammatory reaction they can differentiate into long-lived autoreactive memory cells.

These ideas support a model of three signals being critical for the induction of optimal immunity. Naturally, the first is Ag, the second some type of growth signal such as that from a costimulatory molecule and the third a survival signal, which may be derived from a danger signal. It has been shown that immunity is heightened if T cells are responding in the presence of proinflammatory cytokines. These data lend credence to the three-signal hypothesis, since the same responses are not potent when the third signal is omitted. This theory does not state that this is the only way that immunity can be induced: it states that three signals will potentiate a long-term response. The end result is the accumulation of memory cells.

Acknowledgment. I would like to thank Drs. Rockey and Kerkveilet for careful review of this manuscript. I owe a great deal of gratitude to the members of my laboratory for generating data, reviewing this document and contributing ideas.

REFERENCES

Akbar A. N., Borthwick N. J., Wickremasinghe R. G., Panayoitidis P., Pilling D., Bofill M., Krajewski S., Reed J. C. and Salmon M. (1996): Interleukin-2 receptor common gamma-chain signaling cytokines regulate activated T cell apoptosis in response to growth factor withdrawal: selective induction of anti-apoptotic (bcl-2, bcl-xL) but not pro-apoptotic (bax, bcl-xS) gene expression. Eur. J. Immunol., **26**, 294–299.

Alderson M. R., Armitage R. J., Maraskovsky E., Tough T. W., Roux E., Schooley K., Ramsdell F. and Lynch D. H. (1993): Fas transduces activation signals in normal human T lymphocytes. J. Exp. Med., **178**, 2231–2235.

Anderson G., Hare K. J. and Jenkinson E. J. (1999): Positive selection of thymocytes: the long and winding road. Immunol. Today, **20**, 463–468.

Bernal A., Proft T., Fraser J. D. and Posnett D. N. (1999): Superantigens in human disease. J. Clin. Immunol., **19**, 149–157.

Bretscher P. and Cohn M. (1970): A theory of self-nonself discrimination. Science, **169**, 1042–1049.

Cauley L. S., Cauley K. A., Shub F., Huston G. and Swain S. L. (1997): Transferable anergy: superantigen treatment induces $CD4^+$ T cell tolerance that is reversible and requires $CD4^-CD8^-$ cells and interferon gamma. J. Exp. Med., **186**, 71–81.

Chiller J. M. and Weigle W. O. (1973): Termination of tolerance to human gamma globulin in mice by antigen and bacterial lipopolysaccharide (endotoxin). J. Exp. Med., **137**, 740–750.

Croft M. and Dubey C. (1997): Accessory molecule and costimulation requirements for CD4 T cell response. Crit. Rev. Immunol., **17**, 89–118.

Dresser D. W. (1962): Specific inhibition of antibody production. II. Paralysis induced in adult mice by small quantities of protein antigen. Immunology, **5**, 378–388.

Dresser D. W. and Gowland G. (1964): Immunological paralysis induced in adult rabbits by small amounts of protein antigen. Nature, **203**, 733–736.

Dutton R. W., Bradley L. M. and Swain S. L. (1998): T cell memory. Annu. Rev. Immunol., **16**, 201–223.

Flynn S., Toellner K. M., Raykundalia C., Goodall M. and Lane P. (1998): CD4 T cell cytokine differentiation: the B cell activation molecule, OX40 ligand, instructs CD4 T cells to express interleukin 4 and upregulates expression of the chemokine receptor, Blr-1. J. Exp. Med., **188**, 297–304.

Freund J. (1951): The effect of parafin oil and mycobacteria on antibody formation and sensitization. Am. J. Clin. Pathol., **21**, 645–656.

Gramaglia I., Weinberg A. D., Lemon M. and Croft M. (1998): Ox-40 ligand: a potent costimulatory molecule for sustaining primary CD4 T cell responses. J. Immunol., **161**, 6510–6517.

Gray D. and Matzinger P. (1991): T cell memory is short-lived in the absence of antigen. J. Exp. Med., **174**, 969–974.

Grewal I. S. and Flavell R. A. (1996): The role of CD40 ligand in costimulation and T-cell activation. Immunol. Rev., **153**, 85–106.

Gross J. A., Callas E. and Allison J. P. (1992): Identification and distribution of the costimulatory receptor CD28 in the mouse. J. Immunol., **149**, 380–388.

Guerder S., Picarella D. E., Linsley P. S. and Flavell R. A. (1994): Costimulator B7-1 confers antigen-presenting-cell function to parenchymal tissue and in conjunction with tumor necrosis factor alpha leads to autoimmunity in transgenic mice. Proc. Natl. Acad. Sci. USA, **91**, 5138–5142.

Harding F. A., McArthur J. G., Gross J. A., Raulet D. H. and Allison J. P. (1992): CD28-mediated signalling co-stimulates murine T cells and prevents induction of anergy in T-cell clones. Nature, **356**, 607–609.

Harris N. L. and Ronchese F. (1999): The role of B7 costimulation in T-cell immunity. Immunol. Cell Biol., **77**, 304–311.

Hausmann S. and Wucherpfennig K. W. (1997): Activation of autoreactive T cells by peptides from human pathogens. Curr. Opin. Immunol., **9**, 831–838.

Hou S., Hyland L., Ryan K. W., Portner A. and Doherty P. C. (1994): Virus-specific CD8+ T-cell memory determined by clonal burst size. Nature, **369**, 652–654.

Jenkins M. K., Pardoll D. M., Mitzuguchi J., Chused T. M. and Shwartz R. H. (1987a): Molecular events in the induction of a nonresponsive state in interleukin 2-producing helper T-lymphocyte clones. Proc. Natl. Acad. Sci. USA, **84**, 5409–5413.

Jenkins M. K., Pardoll D. M., Mizuguchi J., Quill H. and Schwartz R. H. (1987b): T cell unresponsiveness *in vivo* and *in vitro*: Fine specificity of induction and molecular characterization of the unresponsive state. Immunol. Rev., **95**, 113–135.

Jenkins M. K. and Schwartz R. H. (1987): Antigen presentation by chemically modified splenocytes induces antigen-specific T cell unresponsiveness *in vitro* and *in vivo*. J. Exp. Med., **165**, 302–319.

Kappler J. W., Roehm N. and Marrack P. (1987): T cell tolerance by clonal elimination in the thymus. Cell, **49**, 273–280.

Kawabe Y. and Ochi A. (1990): Selective anergy of Vβ8+, CD4+ T cells in Staphylococcus enterotoxin-B primed mice. J. Exp. Med., **172**, 1065–1070.

Kawabe Y. and Ochi A. (1991): Programmed cell death and extrathymic reduction of Vbeta8+ CD4+ T cells in mice tolerant to *Staphylococcus aureus* enterotoxin B. Nature, **349**, 245–248.

Kearney E. R., Pape K. A., Loh D. Y. and Jenkins M. K. (1994): Visualization of peptide-specific T cell immunity and peripheral tolerance induction *in vivo*. Immunity, **1**, 327–339.

Kiener P. A., Moran-Davis P., Rankin B. M., Wahl A. F., Aruffo A. and Hollenbaugh D. (1995): Stimulation of CD40 with purified soluble gp39 induces proinflammatory responses in human monocytes. J. Immunol., **155**, 4917–4925.

Kotzin B. L., Leung D. Y., Kappler J. and Marrack P. (1993): Superantigens and their potential role in human disease. Adv. Immunol., **54**, 99–165.

Krammer P. H., Behrmann I., Daniel P., Dhein J. and Debatin K. (1994): Regulation of apoptosis in the immune system. Curr. Opin. Immunol., **6**, 279–289.

Kuroda K., Yagi J., Imanishi K., Yan X.-J., Li X.-Y., Fujimaki W., Kato H., Miyoshi-Akiyama T., Kumazawa Y., Abe H. and Uchiyama T. (1996): Implantation of IL-2-containing osmotic pump prolongs the survival of superantigen-reactive T cells explanded in mice injected with bacterial superantigen. J. Immunol., **157**, 1422–1431.

Lafferty K. J. and Cunningham A. J. (1975): A new analysis of allogeneic interactions. Aust. J. Exp. Biol. Med. Sci., **53**, 27–42.

Lau L. L., Jamieson B. D., Somasundaram T. and Ahmed R. (1994): Cytotoxic T-cell memory without antigen. Nature, **369**, 648–652.

Lenardo M. J. (1991): Interleukin-2 programs mouse αb T lymphocytes for apoptosis. Nature, **353**, 858–861.

Leonard W. J., Noguchi M., Russell S. M. and McBride O. W. (1994): The molecular basis of X-linked severe combined immunodeficiency: the role of the interleukin-2 receptor gamma chain as a common gamma chain, gamma c. Immunol. Rev., **138**, 61–86.

Marrack P., Hugo P., McCormack J. and Kappler J. (1993): Death and T cells. Immunol. Rev., **133**, 119–129.

Marrack P. C. and Kappler J. W. (1990): The staphylococcal enterotoxins and their relatives. Science, **248**, 705–711.

Matzinger P. (1994): Tolerance, danger, and the extended family. Annu. Rev. Immunol., **12**, 991–1045.

Matzinger P. (1998): An innate sense of danger. Semin. Immunol., **10**, 399–415.

Maxwell J. R., Campbell J. D., Kim C. H. and Vella A. T. (1999): CD40 activation boosts T cell immunity *in vivo* by enhancing T cell clonal expansion and delaying peripheral T cell deletion. J. Immunol., **162**, 2024–2034.

Maxwell J. R., Weinberg A., Prell R. A. and Vella A. T. (2000): Danger and OX40 receptor signaling synergize to enhance memory T cell survival by inhibiting peripheral deletion. J. Immunol., **164**, 107–112.

McCormack J. E., Callahan J. E., Kappler J. and Marrack (1993): Profound deletion of mature T cells *in vivo* by chronic exposure to exogenous superantigen. J. Immunol., **150**, 3785–3792.

Melero I., Shuford W. W., Newby S. A., Aruffo A., Ledbetter J. A., Hellstrom K. E., Mittler R. S. and Chen L. (1997): Monoclonal antibodies against the 4-1BB T-cell activation molecule eradicate established tumors. Nat. Med., **3**, 682–685.

Morrissey P. J., Bradley D., Sharrow S. O. and Singer A. (1983): T cell tolerance to non-H-2--encoded stimulatory alloantigens is induced intrathymically but not prethymically. J. Exp. Med., **158**, 365–377.

Mullbacher A. (1994): The long-term maintenance of cytotoxic T cell memory does not require persistence of antigen. J. Exp. Med., **179**, 317–321.

Ohshima Y., Tanaka Y., Tozawa H., Takahashi Y., Maliszewski C. and Delespesse G. (1997): Expression and function of OX40 ligand on human dendritic cells. J. Immunol., **159**, 3838–3848.

Opferman J. T., Ober B. T. and Ashton-Rickardt P. G. (1999): Linear differentiation of cytotoxic effectors into memory T lymphocytes. Science, **283**, 1745–1748.

Paterson D. J., Jefferies W. A., Green J. R., Brandon M. R., Corthesy P., Pullaves M. and

Williams A. F. (1987): Antigens of activated rat T lymphocytes including a molecule of 50,000 Mr detected only on CD4 positive T blasts. Mol. Immunol., **24**, 1281–1290.

Pollok K. E., Kim Y.-J., Zhou Z., Hurtado J., Kim K. K., Pickard R. T. and Kwon B. S. (1993): Inducible T cell antigen 4-1BB. Analysis of expression and function. J. Immunol., **150**, 771–781.

Powell J. D., Ragheb J. A., Kitagawa-Sakakida S. and Schwartz R. H. (1998): Molecular regulation of interleukin-2 expression by CD28 co-stimulation and anergy. Immunol. Rev., **165**, 287–300.

Roy M., Aruffo A., Ledbetter J., Linsley P. and Kehry M. (1995): Studies on the interdependence of gp39 and B7 expression and function during antigen-specific immune response. Eur. J. Immunol., **25**, 596–603.

Shahinian A., Pfeffer K., Lee K. P., Kündig T. M., Kishihara K., Wakeham A., Kawai K., Ohashi P. M., Thompson C. B. and Mak T. W. (1993): Differential T cell costimulatoryr equirements in CD28-deficient mice. Science, **261**, 609–612.

Shuford W. W., Klussman K., Titchler D. D., Loo D. K., Chalupny J., Siadak A. W., Brown T. J., Emswiler J., Raecho H., Larsen C. P., Pearson T. C., Ledbetter J. A., Aruffo A. and Mittler R. S. (1997): 4-1BB constimulatory signals preferentially induce $CD8^+$ T cell proliferation and lead to the amplification *in vivo* of cytotoxic T cell responses. J. Exp. Med., **186**, 47–55.

Sprent J., Lo D., Gao E.-K. and Ron Y. (1998): T cell selection in the thymus. Immunol. Rev., **101**, 173–190.

Stuber E., Neurath M., Calderhead D., Fell H. P. and Strober W. (1995): Cross-linking of OX40 ligand, a member of the TNF/NGF cytokine family, induces proliferation and differentiation in murine splenic B cells. Immunity, **2**, 507–521.

Swain S. L. (1994): Generation and *in vivo* persistence of polarized Th1 and Th2 memory cells. Immunity, **1**, 543–552.

Takahashi C., Mittler R. S. and Vella A. T. (1999): Cutting edge: 4-1BB is a bona fide CD8 T cell survival signal. J. Immunol., **162**, 5037–5040.

Taneja V. and David C. S. (1999): HLA class II transgenic mice as models of human diseases. Immunol. Rev., **169**, 67–79.

Teague T. K., Kappler J. W., Marrack P. and Vella A. T. (1997): Interleukin-6 inhibits resting T cells from apoptosis. J. Immunol., **158**, 5791–5796.

Vella A. T., Dow S., Potter T. A., Kappler J. and Marrack P. (1998): Cytokine-induced survival of activated T cells *in vitro* and *in vivo*. Proc. Natl. Acad. Sci. USA, **95**, 3810–3815.

Vella A. T., McCormack J. E., Linsley P. S., Kappler J. W. and Marrack P. (1995): Lipopolysaccharide interferes with the induction of peripheral T cell death. Immunity, **2**, 261–270.

Vella A. T., Mitchell T., Groth B., Linsley P. S., Green J. M., Thompson C. B., Kappler J. W. and Marrack P. (1997a): CD28 engagement and proinflammatory cytokines contribute to T cell expansion and long-term survival *in vivo*. J. Immunol., **158**, 4714–4720.

Vella A. T., Scherer M. T., Schultz L., Kappler J. W. and Marrack P. (1996): B cells are not essential for peripheral T cell tolerance. Proc. Natl. Acad. Sci. USA, **93**, 951–955.

Vella A., Teague T. K., Ihle J., Kappler J. and Marrack P. (1997b): Interleukin 4 (IL-4) or IL-7 prevents the death of resting T cells: stat6 is probably not required for the effect of IL-4. J. Exp. Med., **186**, 325–330.

Villegas E. N., Elloso M. M., Reichmann G., Peach R. and Hunter C. A. (1999): Role of CD28 in the generation of effector and memory responses required for resistance to toxoplasma gondii. J. Immunol., **163**, 3344–3353.

Vinay D. S. and Kwon B. S. (1998): Role of 4-1BB in immune responses. Semin. Immunol., **10**, 481–489.

Wahl S. M. (1994): Transforming growth factor beta: the good, the bad, and the ugly. J. Exp. Med., **180**, 1587–1590.

Weinberg A. D., Vella A. T. and Croft M. (1998): OX-40: life beyond the effector T cell stage. Semin. Immunol., **10**, 471–480.

Weiner H. L. (1997): Oral tolerance for the treatment of autoimmune diseases. Annu. Rev. Med., **48**, 341–351.

Yssel H., Fasler S., Lamb J. and de Vries J. E. (1994): Induction of non-responsiveness in human allergen-specific type 2 T helper cells. Curr. Opin. Immunol., **6**, 847–852.

Zheng L., Fisher G., Miller R. E., Peschon J., Lynch D. H. and Lenardo M. J. (1995): Induction of apoptosis in mature T cells by tumour necrosis factor. Nature, **377**, 348–351.

Zinkernagel R. M., Planz O., Ehl S., Battegay M., Odermatt B., Klenerman P. and Hengartner H. (1999): General and specific immunosuppression caused by antiviral T-cell responses. Immunol. Rev., **168**, 305–315.

THE PHYSIOLOGICAL ROLE OF REGULATORY T CELLS IN THE PREVENTION OF AUTOIMMUNITY: GENERATION, SPECIFICITY AND MODE OF ACTION

BENEDICT SEDDON

Division of Molecular Immunology, National Institute for Medical Research, London, NW7 1AA UK

Abstract Until recently, the traditional view was that tolerance to self antigens was maintained by a combination of physical deletion, in the thymus, and functional deletion, in the periphery, of autoreactive T cells. There is now, however, abundant evidence that the normal T cell repertoire contains overtly autoreactive T cells whose pathogenic potential is held in check by the activity of a distinct subset of peripheral T cells, the so-called regulatory or suppressor T cells. This article examines data from one model of rodent autoimmunity, where autoimmune pathology develops following thymectomy and irradiation of normal laboratory rats, which characterize the development and function of these so-called regulatory T cells.

Key words: regulatory T cells; autoimmunity; prevention.

1. INTRODUCTION – PASSIVE AND ACTIVE MECHANISMS OF SELF TOLERANCE

The immune system has evolved a number of potent mechanisms for the elimination of foreign pathogens. Given that these effector mechanisms are potentially damaging to the host, an essential feature of the adaptive immune system is its ability to distinguish self antigens from non-self and respond only to the latter. For the most part, the immune system successfully makes this distinction and remains self-tolerant. However, under certain circumstances and in genetically susceptible individuals, failures do occur and the resulting immunopathology can affect a wide variety of tissues, causing

A. Górski et al. (eds.), Autoimmunity, 27–38.

a number of different diseases. Diabetes, arthritis and multiple sclerosis are examples of diseases in which an autoimmune mechanism has been implicated in their pathogenesis.

With regard to T cell tolerance, the immune system has evolved a number of strategies for preventing autoreactive T cells from making potentially pathogenic responses against host tissues. The traditional view holds that T cell self tolerance is maintained by a combination of T cell deletion intrathymically and anergy or indifference extrathymically. During T cell development in the thymus, T cells bearing receptors which recognise complexes of major histocompatibility antigens and self peptides with a high affinity are induced to die (Kappler et al., 1987). In the periphery, foreign antigen is presented to specific T cells by antigen-presenting cells which can provide important co--stimulatory signals for T cell activation, while it is considered that self antigens are presented by cells lacking the ability to provide such signals (Mueller et al., 1989; Nickoloff and Turka, 1994), with the result that potentially autoreactive T cells are either rendered anergic (Mueller et al., 1989) or simply do not respond to antigen (Ohashi et al., 1991). These are passive mechanisms, because they rely upon a functional absence of autoreactive cells, either through their physical deletion intrathymically or their functional inability peripherally. However, it is now clear that these mechansims do not completely account for immunological self tolerance and that other active mechanisms operate, called so because they rely on the regulatory action of T cells upon overtly autoreactive T cells which have neither been deleted nor are anergic. This article reviews data largely from one rodent model of autoimmunity which characterizes the function of these regulatory T cells (T_{reg}). A more detailed analysis of evidence for the existence of regulatory T cells in different models of autoimmunity can be found elsewhere (Saoudi et al., 1996b).

2. EVIDENCE FOR THE EXISTENCE OF T_{REG} IN THE NORMAL T CELL REPERTOIRE

The fact that the normal T cell repertoire contains overtly autoreactive T cells which have not been deleted intrathymically or are anergic has been demonstrated in a variety of rat and mouse models. Rodents that are either congenitally lymphopoenic, such as the BB rat (Crisa et al., 1992), or have been induced to be so by neonatal thymectomy (Sakaguchi et al., 1982) or adult thymectomy and irradiation (Penhale et al., 1973) have been shown to spontaneously develop organ-specific autoimmunity in a strain-dependent manner. Were self tolerance maintained exclusively by a combination of physical and functional deletion of autoreactive cells, a reduction in the size of the T cell pool would not be expected to result in the overt autoimmunity observed in these cases.

In one of these models, normal laboratory rats, with no predisposition to development of spontaneous autoimmunity, could be induced to develop a range of organ-specific autoimmune pathologies when thymectomized between 3 and 6 weeks of age and given 4 doses of irradiation at two-week intervals starting two weeks after thymectomy (TxX protocol hereon) (Penhale et al., 1975). Shortly after the final irradiation, PVG-strain rats developed thyroiditis characterized by high titres of anti-thyroglobulin autoantibody and extensive infiltrates of the thyroid glands (Penhale et al., 1975). PVG.$RT1^u$ rats, which share the same major histocompatibility complex (MHC) haplotype as the spontaneously diabetic BB rat (Crisa et al., 1992), similarly thymectomised and irradiated spontaneously developed a fatal diabetes shortly after the final irradiation (Fowell and Mason, 1993). In a more extreme example, Lewis rats treated in the same way developed a fatal autoimmune pathology involving multiple organs so severe that many rats failed to survive the complete thymectomy and irradiation protocol (Penhale et al., 1973).

Evidence that autoimmunity developed as a result of a failure of T_{reg} to control autoreactive T cells in these rats first came from the observation that disease development could be prevented in some TxX rats following adoptive transfer, shortly after the last irradiation, of splenocytes from normal syngeneic donors (Penhale et al., 1976). Later studies purified and tested the ability of different lymphocyte subsets to prevent autoimmune diabetes in TxX PVG. $RT1^u$ rats and determined that only a specific subset of $CD4^+$ T lymphocytes was capable of preventing disease development upon adoptive transfer. The regulatory T cell population was found amongst $CD4^+$ $TCR\alpha\beta^+$ T cells that express the RT6 antigen but fail to express the CD45 isoform that utilises the C exon (CD45RC), and they were long-lived cells, since they were present in long-term thymectomised rats (Fowell and Mason, 1993). While adoptive transfer of 10^7 $CD4^+$ T cells could only prevent diabetes in 50% of TxX PVG. $RT1^u$ recipients, all recipients of 5×10^6 $CD4^+TCR\alpha\beta^+CD45RC^-$ T cells were protected from disease development, whereas no recipients of $CD4^+TCR\alpha\beta^+CD45RC^+$ T cells were protected (Fowell and Mason, 1993). These data demonstrated that the normal T cell repertoire contains both overtly autoreactive T cells and a phenotypically distinct population of T_{reg} that could control their pathogenic activity.

3. THE ROLE OF THE THYMUS IN THE GENERATION OF T_{REG}

The phenotype of the peripheral T cell subset that contains the T_{reg} ($CD4^+RT6^+CD45RC^-$) is also the phenotype of a resting antigen-experienced cell (Powrie and Mason, 1989). The implication of this result was that T_{reg} are generated in the periphery by clonal expansion of naive cells following encounter with a specific antigen. It was therefore significant to find that $CD4^+CD8^-$ thymocytes, a naive population, are capable of protecting a significant proportion of TxX recipients from development of autoimmunity. This protection was shown to be mediated by mature L-selectin$^+$ $CD4^+CD8^-$ thymocytes and not by a peripheral cell that had recirculated to the thymus (Seddon et al., 1996). Furthermore, the relative potency of $CD4^+CD8^-$ thymocytes in preventing development of autoimmunity is far greater than that of peripheral $CD4^+CD45RC^-$ cells. In thyroiditis development in TxX PVG rats (Seddon and Mason, 1999b) and diabetes in TxX PVG. $RT1^u$ rats (Saoudi et al., 1996a), thymocytes were shown in both cases to be effective at cell doses approximately a tenth of the number of peripheral T cells required. Significantly, this functional potency of $CD4^+CD8^-$ thymocytes appears to be restricted only to their ability to prevent diabetes upon adoptive transfer. When assayed for their ability to provide primed B cells with help for antigen-specific secondary antibody responses, $CD4^+CD8^-$ thymocytes were relatively poor at providing such help in contrast to either naive or primed peripheral $CD4^+$ T cells (Saoudi et al., 1996a).

Together, these data suggest that, rather than being generated by clonal expansion in the periphery, the cells responsible for protection of TxX rats from development of diabetes are already generated at a high frequency in the thymus, and it is for this reason that $CD4^+CD8^-$ thymocytes are such a potent source of T_{reg}. That the thymus is implicated in the generation of T_{reg} that prevent autoimmunity is also suggested by studies of transplantation tolerance in chickens that revealed a potent ability of xenogeneic thymic epithelium to induce tolerance to donor-type grafts. Chicken embryos grafted with quail thymic epithelium (TE) were found to be tolerant to quail limb-bud grafts (Le Douarin et al., 1996). Tolerance was not a consequence of clonal deletion on quail TE, since it was found even in chicks in which some of the thymic lobes were entirely of chick origin. The implication of these data is that the selection of T cells on foreign TE generates T_{reg} that maintain dominant tolerance to grafts of the donor genotype. It is therefore significant that expression of mRNA for many so-called tissue-specific antigens can be detected in the thymus, including insulin, thyroglobulin and myelin basic protein, all of which have been implicated as autoantigens (Antonia et al., 1995; Heath et al., 1998;

Morahan et al., 1989). Taken together, these data support the view that selection of the T cell repertoire on self peptides may be important in generating T_{reg}.

4. DEVELOPMENT OF T_{REG} REQUIRES RELEVENT EXTRATHYMIC SELF ANTIGEN

While there is strong evidence that the thymus plays a vital role in generating T_{reg}, the observation that the T_{reg} in the periphery shares the phenotype of an antigen-experienced cell suggests that the development of functional T_{reg} from thymic precursors requires encounter with specific antigen which drives maturation. Evidence that extrathymic antigen is required for this process comes from studies of rats whose thyroid glands were ablated *in utero*.

In the first series of studies, athyroid rats were generated by exposure of rats *in utero* to radioactive ^{131}I at day 17–18 of gestation, just as the embryonic thyroids become able to concentrate iodine and, significantly, prior to population of the periphery with mature T cells. Syngeneic thyroid grafts in athyroid rats underwent rapid rejection with extensive leukocytic infiltration, whereas third-party endocrine organ grafts were unaffected (Eishi and McCullagh, 1988a). Significantly, when athyroid rats were parabiosed with euthyroid partners, the athyroid rats accepted thyroid grafts (McCullagh, 1990), suggesting that euthyroid rats provided T_{reg}, lacking in the athyroid partner, that could prevent thyroid graft rejection.

A second study provides further evidence that athyroid rats specifically lack T_{reg} that prevent thyroid autoimmunity. When $CD4^+$ T cells were obtained from athyroid PVG rats, it was found that these cells, unlike those from euthyroid donors, were unable to prevent thyroiditis upon adoptive transfer into TxX recipient rats (Seddon and Mason, 1999a). The deficit in T_{reg} activity is specific for thyroid antigens, since $CD4^+$ T cells from athyroid PVG.RT1^u donors retain the ability to prevent diabetes upon adoptive transfer into prediabetic TxX PVG.RT1^u rats. Significantly, $CD4^+$ single positive thymocytes from athyroid donors are still able to prevent disease upon adoptive transfer. This result implies that intrathymic development of T_{reg} precursors is normal in these rats and that the failure to develop specific T_{reg} in the periphery is due entirely to the absence of the specific peripheral autoantigen.

The precise role of peripheral autoantigen in generating T_{reg} is not clear from these studies. It is not possible from these data to determine whether athyroid rats fail to expand thyroid-specific T_{reg} to a sufficient frequency required for activity or whether these cells simply fail to survive in the absence of relevant autoantigen. The dependence on peripheral antigen for the development of T_{reg} may explain the finding that the balance between autoreactive and regulatory T cells is a very fine one (Saoudi et al., 1996), with the number of T_{reg} found in the periphery only just sufficient to prevent autoimmunity. The implication of this result is that generation of T_{reg} in the periphery is under homeostatic control, such that only as many T_{reg} are generated as are required following encounter with relevant peripheral self antigen. This could also explain the relative differences in the potency of thymocytes and peripheral T cells in preventing autoimmunity. Thymocytes contain a high frequency of T_{reg} precursors which, under conditions of T_{reg} depravition found in lymphopoenic TxX rats, can all be recruited to the T_{reg} pool, whereas peripheral T cells only contain a fixed number of terminally differentiated T_{reg}, with no further recruitment possible. This difference in the plasticity of the two populations could explain the differences in their potency.

It is not known what might regulate this homeostasis; transient activation of autoreactive T cells may drive maturation of T_{reg}, and it is also possible that T_{reg} themselves regulate their own development by inhibiting further T_{reg} generation when they are at a sufficiently high frequency. The advantage of such mechanisms is that they ensure that the immune system is not overly populated by T_{reg}, which could interfere with the ability of the immune system to mount a normal response to a foreign pathogen.

5. MODE OF ACTION OF T_{REG}

Data that contribute to an understanding of how T_{reg} function in this system comes from both *in vitro* and *in vivo* studies. Studies of subsets of $CD4^+$ T cells as defined by their expression of CD45RC have provided some clues. $CD4^+CD45RC^+$ T cells bear some of the characteristics of Th1-like cells, since they secrete high levels of IFN-γ and IL-2 following activation *in vitro* (Arthur and Mason, 1986; McKnight et al., 1991), but, more significantly, there is evidence that they contain cells with an autoreactive potential, since their adoptive transfer into nude recipients results in a wasting disease characterized by mononuclear infiltrates in many organs (Powrie and Mason, 1990). In contrast, $CD4^+CD45RC^-$ cells, which contain the T_{reg} population, are a potent source of IL-4 following activation *in vitro* (McKnight et al., 1991) and their co-transfer with $CD4^+CD45RC^+$ cells into nude recipients prevents the induction of wasting disease by the latter population (Powrie and Mason, 1990). The most direct interpretation of these data are that Th2 cytokine-secreting T_{reg} counteract the activity of Th1-like autoreactive T cells. While, for many years, this had been an attractive model for the function of T_{reg} in several systems, data from more recent studies suggest this interpretation is at best an oversimplification.

As described earlier, TxX PVG.RT1^u rats spontaneously developed insulin-dependent diabetes mellitus, while PVG rats subjected to the same protocol developed autoimmune thyroiditis. Diabetes in PVG. RT1^u rats is characterized by a cell-mediated immunopathology, dependent on the cytolytic activity of CD8$^+$ T cells (Fowell and Mason, 1993). In contrast, the thyroiditis that develops in PVG rats occurs independently of CD8$^+$ T cells and is characterised by extensive plasma cell infiltration of the thyroids and high titres of anti-thyroglobulin antibodies of the Th2-associated IgG1 but little of the Th1-associated IgG2b isotype (Seddon and Mason, 1999b). That autoimmune thyroiditis represents a Th2-mediated immunopathology is further supported by the observation that PVG rats immunized with homologous thyroglobulin in complete Freunds adjuvant, an adjuvant that strongly promotes Th1-responses, developed high titres of Th1-associated IgG isotype anti-thyroglobulin antibodies (Seddon and Mason, 1999b), but failed to develop thyroiditis (Eishi and McCullagh, 1988b). Given the stark contrast in the pathogenesis of diabetes and thyroiditis in these TxX rats, it is highly significant that both diseases were prevented by their reconstitution with the same subset of T cells. In both instances, rats reconstituted with either CD4$^+$CD45RC$^-$ peripheral T cells or CD4$^+$CD8$^-$ thymocytes were protected from development of disease (Saoudi et al., 1996a; Seddon and Mason, 1999b). These data do not, therefore, support the view that the mechanism of regulation involves a switch from a Th1- to Th2-like response, but rather depends on the specific suppression of autoreactive T cells.

Studies using neutralising antibodies against cytokines provide data implicating specific cytokines in the mechanism of regulation by T_{reg} in TxX rats. IL-4 and TGF-β both appear to be essential for the prevention of thyroiditis by thymocytes and peripheral cells, since neutralization of one or the other cytokine is sufficent to abrogate protection (Seddon and Mason, 1999b). While these data indicate the requirement for these cytokines, no conclusion can be drawn with regard to where and by what cell type they are made or the target of their activity. However, the immuno-suppressive effect of TGF-β has been reported in a number of systems (Han et al., 1996; Kulkarni et al., 1993; Miller et al., 1992; Shull et al., 1992; Weiner et al., 1994) and has been implicated in suppression of both cell-mediated responses, as in models of inflammatory bowel disease (Powrie et al., 1996) and in humoral autoimmunity induced by mercuric chloride (Bridoux et al., 1997). The role of IL-4 in T_{reg} function is less clear. The ability of IL-4 to modulate immune responses from pro-inflammatory Th1 to anti-inflammatory Th2 responses may explain its protective effects in some autoimmune systems (Mueller et al., 1996; Rapoport et al., 1993). However, data from other studies implicate a role for IL-4 in the generation of T_{reg}, since IL-4 has been shown to promote TGF-β production *in vitro* (Seder et al., 1998), while administration of IL-4 *in vivo* synergises with sub-optimal doses of orally administered antigen to induce oral tolerance, a process also shown to be TGF-β dependent (Inobe et al., 1996; 1998). Taken together, these data suggest that IL-4 may have a role as a growth factor in the generation of T_{reg}, while the role of TGF-β is as an effector cytokine, effecting both T cells and modulating antigen-presenting cell function (Ria et al., 1998; Seder et al., 1998).

6. A MODEL FOR T_{REG} DEVELOPMENT AND FUNCTION

While the data reviewed in this article still leave many questions unanswered, it is possible to propose a model of T_{reg} development and function

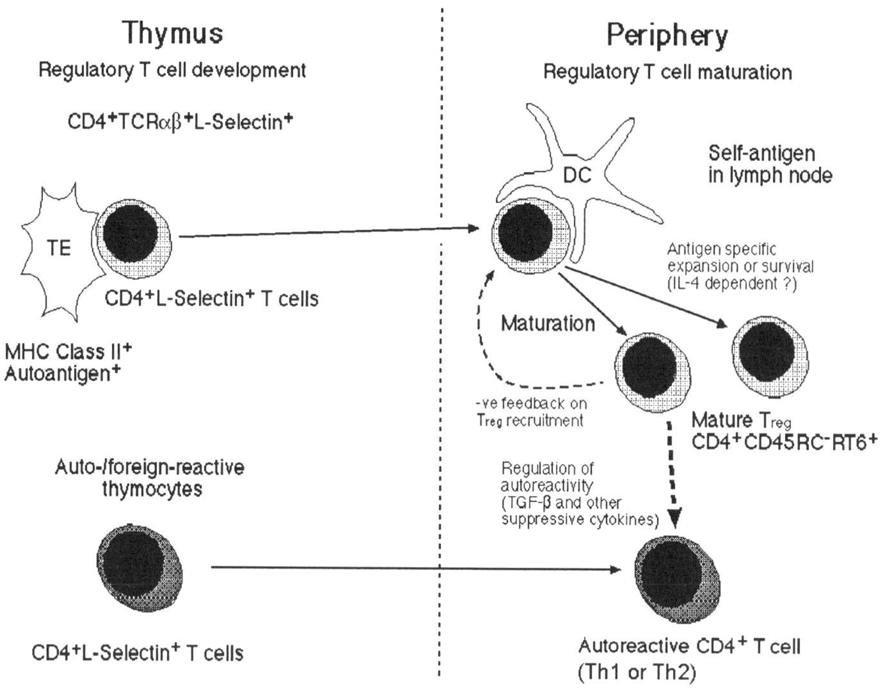

Figure 1. Model of T_{reg} development in rats. The figure summarizes current knowledge of the developmental pathway of T_{reg} in rats, from positive selection in the thymus to final maturation into an effector state in the periphery. Solid arrows indicate T cell development, while dashed arrows indicate the action of T_{reg} either on autoreactive T cells or as part of a homeostatic feedback regulation to prevent excessive generation of T_{reg}. Abbreviations: TE – thymic epithelium, DC – dendritic cell, MHC – major histocompatibility complex, T_{reg} – regulatory T cells, -ve – negative

(Fig. 1). In this model, selection of the T cell repertoire in the thymus on self determinants not only generates the precursors of naïve T cells that will recognise and respond to foreign determinants, but also programs cells with the potential to become regulatory T cells. The signal required for completion of maturation comes in the periphery only if appropriate self antigen is encountered by T_{reg} precursors. This peripheral selection event is either permissive for T_{reg} survival or may drive expansion of T_{reg}, a process possibly dependent on IL-4. Finally, T_{reg} function to specifically suppress Th1 and Th2 autoreactive T cells through the secretion of TGF-β and, most likely, other cytokines, such as IL-10, which have been implicated in T_{reg} function in other systems (Groux and Powrie, 1999).

REFERENCES

Antonia S. J., Geiger T., Miller J. and Flavell R. A. (1995): Mechanisms of immune tolerance induction through the thymic expression of a peripheral tissue-specific protein. Int Immunol., **7**, 715–725.

Arthur R. P. and Mason D. (1986): T cells that help B cell responses to soluble antigen are distinguishable from those producing interleukin 2 on mitogenic or allogeneic stimulation. J. Exp. Med., **163**, 774–786.

Bridoux F., Badou A., Saoudi A., Bernard I., Druet E., Pasquier R., Druet P. and Pelletier L. (1997): Transforming growth factor beta (TGF-beta)-dependent inhibition of T helper cell 2 (Th2)-induced autoimmunity by self-major histocompatibility complex (MHC) class II-specific, regulatory CD4(+) T cell lines. J. Exp. Med., **185**, 1769–1775.

Crisa L., Mordes J. P. and Rossini A. A. (1992): Autoimmune diabetes mellitus in the BB rat. Diabetes Metab. Rev., **8**, 4–37.

Eishi Y. and McCullagh P. (1988a): Acquisition of immunological self-recognition by the fetal rat. Immunology, **64**, 319–323.

Eishi Y. and McCullagh P. (1988b): PVG rats, resistant to experimental allergic thyroiditis, develop high serum levels of thyroglobulin after sensitization. Clin. Immunol. Immunopathol., **49**, 101–106.

Fowell D. and Mason D. (1993): Evidence that the T cell repertoire of normal rats contains cells with the potential to cause diabetes. Characterization of the CD4+ T cell subset that inhibits this autoimmune potential. J. Exp. Med., **177**, 627–636.

Groux H. and Powrie F. (1999): Regulatory T cells and inflammatory bowel disease. Immunol. Today, **20**, 442–445.

Han H. S., Jun H. S., Utsugi T. and Yoon J. W. (1996): A new type of CD4+ suppressor T cell completely prevents spontaneous autoimmune diabetes and recurrent diabetes in syngeneic islet-transplanted NOD mice. J. Autoimmun., **9**, 331–339.

Heath V. L., Moore N. C., Parnell S. M. and Mason D. W. (1998): Intrathymic expression of genes involved in organ specific autoimmune disease. J. Autoimmun., **11**, 309–318.

Inobe J. I., Chen Y. and Weiner H. L. (1996): *In vivo* administration of IL-4 induces TGF-beta--producing cells and protects animals from experimental autoimmune encephalomyelitis. Ann. NY Acad. Sci., **778**, 390–392.

Inobe J., Slavin A. J., Komagata Y., Chen Y., Liu L. and Weiner H. L. (1998): IL-4 is a differentiation factor for transforming growth factor-beta secreting Th3 cells and oral administration of IL-4 enhances oral tolerance in experimental allergic encephalomyelitis. Eur. J. Immunol., **28**, 2780–2790.

Kappler J. W., Roehm M. and Marrack P. (1987): T cell tolerance by clonal elimination in the thymus. Cell, **49**, 273–280.

Kulkarni A. B., Huh C. G., Becker D., Geiser A., Lyght M., Flanders K. C., Roberts A. B., Sporn M. B., Ward J. M. and Karlsson S. (1993): Transforming growth factor beta 1 null mutation in mice causes excessive inflammatory response and early death. Proc. Natl. Acad. Sci. USA, **90**, 770–774.

Le Douarin N., Corbel C., Bandeira A., Thomas-Vaslin V., Modigliani Y., Coutinho A. and Salaün J. (1996): Evidence for a thymus-dependent form of tolerance that is not based on elimination or anergy of reactive T cells. Immunol. Rev., **149**, 35–54.

McCullagh P. (1990): Curtailment of autoimmunity following parabiosis with a normal partner. Immunology, **71**, 595–597.

McKnight A. J., Barclay A. N. and Mason D. W. (1991): Molecular cloning of rat interleukin 4 cDNA and analysis of the cytokine repertoire of subsets of $CD4^+$ T cells. Eur. J. Immunol., **21**, 1187–1194.

Miller A., Lider O., Roberts A. B., Sporn M. B. and Weiner H. L. (1992): Suppressor T cells generated by oral tolerization to myelin basic protein suppress both *in vitro* and *in vivo* immune responses by the release of transforming growth factor beta after antigen-specific triggering. Proc. Natl. Acad. Sci. USA, **89**, 421–425.

Morahan G., Allison J. and Miller J. F. (1989): Tolerance of class I histocompatibility antigens expressed extrathymically. Nature, **339**, 622–624.

Mueller D. L., Jenkins M. K. and Schwartz R. H. (1989): Clonal expansion versus functional clonal inactivation: a costimulatory signalling pathway determines the outcome of T cell antigen receptor occupancy. Annu. Rev. Immunol., **7**, 445–480.

Mueller R., Krahl T. and Sarvetnick N. (1996): Pancreatic expression of interleukin-4 abrogates insulitis and autoimmune diabetes in nonobese diabetic (NOD) mice. J. Exp. Med., **184**, 1093–1099.

Nickoloff B. J. and Turka L. A. (1994): Immunological functions of non-professional antigen--presenting cells: new insights from studies of T-cell interactions with keratinocytes. Immunol. Today, **15**, 464–469.

Ohashi P. S., Oehen S., Buerki K., Pircher H., Ohashi C. T., Odermatt B., Malissen B., Zinkernagel R. M. and Hengartner H. (1991): Ablation of "tolerance" and induction of diabetes by virus infection in viral antigen transgenic mice. Cell, **65**, 305–317.

Penhale W. J., Farmer A. and Irvine W. J. (1975): Thyroiditis in T cell-depleted rats. Influence of strain, radiation dose, adjuvants and antilymphocyte serum. Clin. Exp. Immunol., **21**, 362–375.

Penhale W. J., Farmer A., McKenna R. P. and Irvine W. J. (1973): Spontaneous thyroiditis in thymectomized and irradiated Wistar rats. Clin. Exp. Immunol., **15**, 225–236.

Penhale W. J., Irvine W. J., Inglis J. R. and Farmer A. (1976): Thyroiditis in T cell-depleted rats: suppression of the autoallergic response by reconstitution with normal lymphoid cells. Clin. Exp. Immunol., **25**, 6–16.

Powrie F., Carlino J., Leach M. W., Mauze S. and Coffman R. L. (1996): A critical role for transforming growth factor-β but not interleukin 4 in the suppression of T helper type 1-mediated colitis by CD45RB low CD4+ T cells. J. Exp. Med., **183**, 2669–2674.

Powrie F. and Mason D. (1989): The MRC OX-22- CD4+ T cells that help B cells in secondary immune responses derive from naive precursors with the MRC OX-22+ CD4+ phenotype. J. Exp. Med., **169**, 653–662.

Powrie F. and Mason D. (1990): OX-22high CD4+ T cells induce wasting disease with multiple organ pathology: prevention by the OX-22low subset (published erratum appears in J. Exp. Med. 1991 Apr 1;173(4), 1037). J. Exp. Med., **172**, 1701–1708.

Rapoport M. J., Jaramillo A., Zipris D., Lazarus A. H., Serreze D. V., Leiter E. H., Cyopick P., Danska J. S. and Delovitch T. L. (1993): Interleukin 4 reverses T cell proliferative unresponsiveness and prevents the onset of diabetes in nonobese diabetic mice. J. Exp. Med., **178**, 87–99.

Ria F., Penna G. and Adorini L. (1998): Th1 cells induce and Th2 inhibit antigen-dependent IL-12 secretion by dendritic cells. Eur. J. Immunol., **28**, 2003–2016.

Sakaguchi S., Takahashi T. and Nishizuka Y. (1982): Study on cellular events in post-thymectomy autoimmune oophoritis in mice. II. Requirements of Lyt-1 cells in normal female mice for the prevention of oophoritis. J. Exp. Med., **156**, 1577–1586.

Saoudi A., Seddon B., Fowell D. and Mason D. (1996a): The thymus contains a high frequency of cells that prevent autoimmune diabetes on transfer into pre-diabetic recipients. J. Exp. Med., **184**, 2393–2398.

Saoudi A., Seddon B., Heath V., Fowell V. and Mason D. (1996b): The physiological role of regulatory T cells in the prevention of autoimmunity: the function of the thymus in the generation of the regulatory T cell subset. Immunol. Rev., **149**, 195–216.

Seddon B. and Mason D. (1999a): Peripheral autoantigen induces regulatory T cells that prevent autoimmunity. J. Exp. Med., **189**, 877–881.

Seddon B. and Mason D. (1999b): Regulatory T cells in the control of autoimmunity: the essential role of TGF-β and IL-4 in the prevention of autoimmune thyroiditis in rats by peripheral CD4+CD45RC- cells and CD4+CD8- thymocytes. J. Exp. Med., **189**, 279–288.

Seddon B., Saoudi A., Nicholson M. and Mason D. (1996): CD4+CD8- thymocytes that express L-Selectin protect rats from diabetes upon adoptive transfer. Eur. J. Immunol., **26**, 2702–2708.

Seder R. A., Marth T., Sieve M. C., Strober W., Letterio J. J., Roberts A. B. and Kelsall B. (1998): Factors involved in the differentiation of TGF-beta-producing cells from naive CD4+ T cells: IL-4 and IFN-gamma have opposing effects, while TGF-beta positively regulates its own production. J. Immunol., **160**, 5719–5728.

Shull M. M., Ormsby I., Kier A. B., Pawlowski S., Diebold R. J., Yin M., Allen R., Sidman C., Proetzel G., Calvin D., Annunziata N. and Doetschman T. (1992): Targeted disruption of the mouse transforming growth factor-β1 gene results in multifocal inflammatory disease. Nature, **359**, 693–699.

Weiner H. L., Friedman A., Miller A., Khoury S. J., al-Sabbagh A., Santos L., Sayegh M., Nussenblatt R. B., Trentham D. E. and Hafler D. A. (1994): Oral tolerance: immunologic mechanisms and treatment of animal and human organ-specific autoimmune diseases by oral administration of autoantigens. Annu. Rev. Immunol., **12**, 809–837.

EPITOPE SPREADING: A MECHANISM FOR PROGRESSION OF AUTOIMMUNE DISEASE

VINCENT K. TUOHY[1, 2] and R. PHILIP KINKEL[2]

[1] *Department of Immunology, Lerner Research Institute, The Cleveland Clinic Foundation, Cleveland, OH, USA*
[2] *Mellen Center for Multiple Sclerosis Research and Treatment, Department of Neurology, The Cleveland Clinic Foundation, Cleveland, OH, USA*

Abstract Autoimmune diseases are typically characterized by a persistent inflammatory self-recognition process that ultimately leads to chronic progressive disability. Over the past several years we have addressed the fundamental question of why autoimmune diseases are chronic. Our working hypothesis in these studies has been that autoimmunity involves a continuous acquisition of new self-recognition events, thereby providing an inflammatory steady-state that leads to chronicity. This acquired T cell neoautoreactivity is commonly referred to as epitope spreading. By studying multiple sclerosis (MS) and its related animal model, experimental autoimmune encephalomyelitis (EAE), we have found that chronic progression of autoimmune disease is invariably linked to the development of an epitope-spreading process that manifests as a cascade of inflammatory T cell neoautoreactivities to a sequential series of predictable new target self-antigens. However, our most recent observations indicate that the emergence of epitope spreading is accompanied by a concurrent regression of the established primary autoreactivity associated with disease onset. Thus, our studies indicate that progression of autoimmune disease involves a shifting of T cell autoreactivity from primary initiating self-determinants to defined cascades of secondary determinants that sustain the inflammatory self-recognition process during progression to chronicity. Our data support the view that the natural development of self-recognition during autoimmune disease may best be understood when considered in the temporal context of an "epitope *du jour*" and "moving target" perspective.

Key words: autoimmunity; EAE/MS; T cell; myelin; demyelination.

Abbreviations used: CDMS – clinically definite multiple sclerosis, CNS – central nervous system, EAE – experimental autoimmune encephalomyelitis, IMDS – isolated mono-symptomatic demyelinating syndrome, MBP – myelin basic protein, MOG – myelin oligodendrocyte glycoprotein, MRI – magnetic resonance imaging, MS – multiple sclerosis, PBMC – peripheral blood mononuclear cells, PLP – myelin proteolipid protein, MHC – major histocompatibility complex.

A. Górski et al. (eds.), Autoimmunity, 39–48.

1. INTRODUCTION

Much of our current understanding of self-recognition in multiple sclerosis (MS) stems from studies on experimental autoimmune encephalomyelitis (EAE), an animal model with many clinical and histopathologic similarities to MS (Martin et al., 1992; Steinman, 1996). EAE is induced by immunization of animals with either whole central nervous system (CNS) tissue, myelin or myelin proteins such as myelin basic protein (MBP), myelin proteolipid protein (PLP) or myelin oligodendrocyte glycoprotein (MOG). EAE is mediated by $CD4^+$ T cells of the Th1 phenotype (IL-2, IFN-γ, TNF-β) that recognize peptide determinants of CNS myelin proteins in the context of major histocompatibility complex (MHC) class II molecules and initiate a cascade of events leading ultimately to paralysis accompanied by perivascular mononuclear infiltrates and demyelination in CNS white matter (Martin et al., 1992; Raine, 1984).

SWXJ mice develop a relapsing form of EAE that progresses to chronicity. Following immunization with the immunodominant encephalitogenic determinant PLP 139-151, SWXJ mice develop acute EAE followed by a relapsing-remitting clinical course, with each relapse being progressively more severe and each remission leaving the mice progressively more impaired. Within 4 months after immunization, the majority of SWXJ mice reach a chronic-progressive stage of EAE characterized by a gradual inability to initiate any self-directed movement and by severe CNS demyelination, particularly pronounced in the spinal cord (Sobel et al., 1991; Tuohy and Thomas, 1995).

A growing number of studies indicate that relapse and progression of EAE may be due to the acquisition of T cell responses to new myelin protein determinants during the course of disease. This acquired T cell neoautoreactivity is commonly referred to as epitope or determinant spreading and is presumably due to endogenous priming with new self-antigens presented during the inflammatory destruction of tissue to an infiltrating immune system (Tuohy et al., 1994; Vanderlugt and Miller, 1996). The first definitive report of intramolecular epitope spreading may be attributed to McCarron et al. (1990), who showed that $(SJLxPL)F_1$ mice acquired a new class II MHC-restricted response to MBP during relapse that was not present during the primary inflammatory attack. Lehmann et al. (1992) extended this finding and found that the specificity of the T cell repertoire in $(SJLxB10.PL)F_1$ mice was restricted to the priming immunodominant MBP 1-11 determinant during the inductive phase of MBP--induced EAE, but broadened with increasing time to include reactivity to the MBP cryptic determinants p35-47, p81-100 and p121-140. Most importantly, the observed epitope spreading did not require immunization with whole MBP but occurred even when the priming immunogen was the MBP 1-11 peptide determinant. Shifts in MBP, epitope recognition during the course of EAE have also been observed in SJL/J and B10.PL parental mouse strains (Bhardwaj et al., 1994) and in Lewis rats (Mor and Coher, 1993).

Intermolecular spreading was described by Perry et al. (1991) who showed proliferative responses and delayed-type hypersensitivity to PLP during the course of EAE in (SJLxPL)F_1 mice immunized with MBP. The pathogenicity of intermolecular spreading was established by Cross et al. (1993), who were able to transfer EAE with PLP 139-151 stimulated spleen cells from SJL/J mice that had previously developed passive disease mediated by the immunodominant MBP 87-99 determinant. McRae et al. (1995) showed that progression of PLP 139-151-induced EAE could be inhibited by inducing tolerance to whole PLP after recovery from the primary attack. The induction of tolerance inhibited the development of neoautoreactivity directed toward the encephalitogenic PLP 178-191, thereby providing functional evidence, that epitope spreading is a pathogenic process that may be targeted therapeutically with peptide-specific treatment after disease onset. The following account details our experimental evidence, which provides support for the view that epitope spreading is a pathogenic mechanism for progression to chronicity in autoimmune disease.

2. EPITOPE SPREADING IN EAE

We have systematically assessed the pattern of intra- and intermolecular determinant spreading as a function of time in SWXJ mice immunized with the immunodominant PLP 139-151 (Yu et al., 1996a). We found that the order in which new determinants are recognized during the course of disease follows an ordered, predictable, sequential pattern. After immunization of SWXJ mice with PLP 139-151, a sequential cascade of self-recognition occurred. At 4, 8 and 12 weeks after immunization, responses to PLP 249-273, MBP 87-99 and PLP 178-191, respectively, emerged. Thus, at 12 weeks after priming with PLP 139-151, SWXJ mice consistently showed a chronic accumulation of neurologic deficit accompanied by severe CNS demyelination and a cascading accumulation of neoautoreactivity involving PLP 139-151 → PLP 249-273 → MBP 87-99 → PLP 178-191. Similar patterns of temporally spaced neoautoreactivity were observed following priming of SWXJ mice with other encephalitogenic determinants, including PLP 104-117 and PLP 178-191 (Fig. 1a, b).

In addition, we observed an invariant relationship between the development of relapse/progression and the spreading of self-recognition to new immunodominant encephalitogenic determinants. Moreover, we found that peptide-specific tolerance to spreading, but not to "nonspreading", determinants after disease onset prevents subsequent chronic progression of EAE. Finally, we showed that CD4+ Th1 T cells generated *in vivo* to spreading determinants are autonomously pathogenic, since they adoptively transfer EAE into naive recipients even after photolytic elimination of T cells

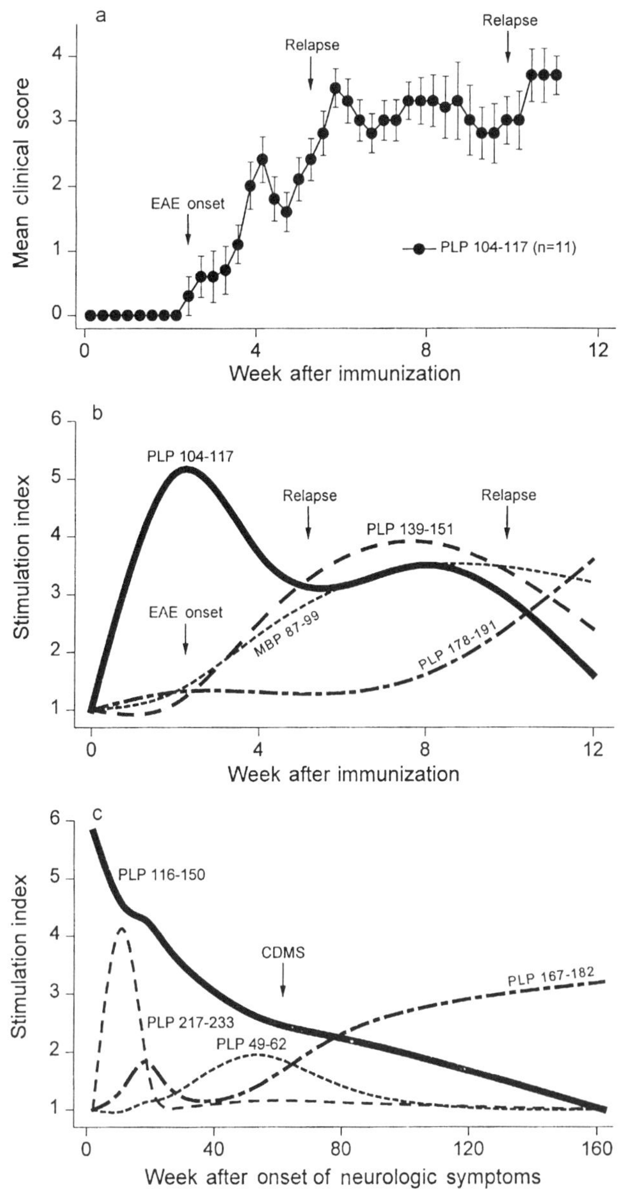

responding to the priming immunogen (Yu et al., 1996b). Thus, our data indicate that determinant spreading is a pathogenic process that leads to relapse and chronic-progression of autoimmune disease, and that the predictable sequential pattern of the determinant-spreading cascade provides a basis for peptide-specific therapy after the onset of clinical disease.

3. EPITOPE SPREADING IN MS

We next asked the question whether epitope spreading occurs during the development and progression of MS (Tuohy et al., 1997). Since MS typically persists for many years before a definitive diagnosis can be made, we focused our studies on patients at the earliest stage of the disease process that ultimately leads to clinically definite MS (CDMS). Patients with isolated monosymptomatic demyelinating syndromes (IMDS) have distinct clinical disorders often associated with the eventual progression to CDMS (Beck et al., 1993; Filippi et al., 1994; Morrissey et al., 1993). By magnetic resonance imaging (MRI) analysis, IMDS patients showing only the CNS lesion responsible for acute symptoms (monocentric monophasic IMDS) are widely viewed to represent the earliest stage at which inflammatory demyelination can be followed from the genuine onset of disease.

Figure 1. The epitope-spreading cascade accompanies progression of EAE and MS: a – immunization of SWXJ mice with PLP 104-117 results in a relapsing-remitting course of EAE that progresses to chronicity. Each relapse is followed by an incomplete recovery that results in a progressive accumulation of neurologic deficit. Similar clinical profiles occur following immunization with PLP 139-151 and PLP 178-191. Error bars show ±SEM; b – a predictable sequential epitope-spreading cascade accompanies progression to chronicity in EAE. Induction of EAE by immunization of SWXJ mice with PLP 104-117 results in a temporally spaced cascade of neoautoreactivity involving PLP 104-117 → PLP 139-151→ MBP 87-99 → PLP 178-191. Similar, and perhaps more pronounced, sequential cascades occur during progression of EAE induced with other encephalitogenic PLP determinants, including PLP 139-151 and PLP 178-191. It should be noted that EAE progression continues long after responses to the priming PLP 104-117 determinant have peaked, regressed, and virtually disappeared. The data are represented as spline curve plots of mean splenocyte proliferative responses of at least three mice tested at each 0, 2, 4, 8 and 12 week time points; c – progression of IMDS → CDMS is accompanied by the spontaneous regression of the proliferative autoreactivity associated with initial IMDS symptoms and by the concurrent emergence of epitope spreading. IMDS patient DL showed IMDS → CDMS progression 60 weeks after the initial onset of IMDS symptoms at week 0. Disease progression involved a sustained neoautoreactivity to PLP 167-182 accompanied by a regression and eventual disappearance of proliferative responses to the PLP 116-150 determinant associated with disease onset. The data are represented as spline curve plots of the mean proliferative responses of PBMC on each day tested

Our approach was to determine serial changes over a 12-18 month period in response to an epitope-mapping series of 265 12-mer PLP peptides by PBMC from IMDS patients. We found that an extensive array of PLP peptides could elicit autoreactivity. Moreover, differential autoreactive patterns were evident within IMDS patient subpopulations distinguished by the absence or presence of old inactive lesions. Monocentric monophasic IMDS patients with no evidence of prior subclinical disease typically showed fully sustained autoreactivity, characterized by extensive plasticity, epitope focusing, shifting and spreading of responses to new self-determinants (Fig. 1c). In contrast, multicentric monophasic IMDS patients with putative evidence of prior asymptomatic lesion formation typically showed partially sustained autoreactivity, characterized by abrupt abrogation of responses to an extensive array of self-determinants. No sustained autoreactivity was observed in normal control subjects or in patients with other neurologic diseases. Our results indicate that self-recognition associated with the development of MS is characterized by autoreactive diversity, plasticity and instability, with epitope spreading being a core manifestation of the observed plasticity.

We have also found that the neoautoreactivity occurring during the progression of MS involves HLA-DP-restricted responses of autoreactive $CD4^+$ T cells (Yu et al., 1998). In our human studies, we have never observed a consensus determinant recognized by patients sharing common HLA-DR and -DQ class II genes, including several study subjects expressing the DRB1*1501/DRB5*0101/DQB1*0602 haplotype associated with increased risk for developing MS (Allen et al., 1994; Francis et al., 1991). However, we did observe epitope spreading to PLP 50-69 in each of two study subjects showing complete disparity at HLA-DR and HLA-DQ but identity at the HLA-DP class II allele DPB1*0301. Upon further analysis we found that peptide-specific proliferation of T cell lines generated from both patients was inhibited by treatment at the initiation of culture with monoclonal antibody specific for HLA-DP, but not with antibody specific for either HLA-DR or -DQ. Moreover, the derived T cell lines showed peptide-specific lytic activity against homozygous-typing B cells expressing the DPB1*0301 class II allele, but not against target cells compatible at HLA-DR and -DQ alleles. Our data indicate that self-presentation by HLA-DP may play an important role in the spreading and propagation of autoreactivity during the clinical progression of MS.

4. REGRESSION, SPREADING, AND PROGRESSION OF AUTOIMMUNE DISEASE

Recently, we have directly addressed the relative roles of primary autoreactivity and secondary epitope spreading in the progression of both EAE and MS. We serially evaluated the development of several epitope-spreading cascades in SWXJ mice primed with distinctly different encephalitogenic PLP determinants and in monophasic monocentric IMDS patients as their disease progressed to CDMS. Our results showed that in both EAE (Fig. 1a, b) and MS (Fig. 1c), primary proliferative autoreactivity associated with onset of clinical disease invariably regressed with time and was often undetectable during periods of disease progression. In contrast, the emergence of sustained secondary autoreactivity to spreading determinants was consistently associated with disease progression in both EAE and MS. Thus, chronic progression of EAE and MS actually involves a definitive shift of autoreactivity from primary initiating self-determinants to defined cascades of secondary determinants that sustain the self-recognition process during disease progression (Tuohy et al., 1999a; 1999b). A shifting, rather than an accumulation, of autoreactivites implies that the T cell repertoire associated with the progression of autoimmune disease is dramatically different from that associated with disease onset. Moreover, it becomes increasingly more difficult to explain how disease progression can result from an undetectable initiating primary autoreactivity.

The repeated failure to demonstrate memory responses to self-determinants indicates that autoimmune memory has features not observed in traditional memory responses to environmental antigens. This apparent anomaly may find some explanation from recent studies that showed complete deletion of the memory repertoire to viral antigens following high-load inoculation with virus (Gallimore et al., 1998). A similar outcome seems feasible in autoimmunity when one considers the virtually infinite antigen load of constantly synthesized self-proteins. Thus, chronic self-stimulation may result in T cell exhaustion and the peripheral apoptotic deletion of the autoreactive repertoire associated with disease onset, leaving only the developing, endogenously primed neoautoreactive repertoire to sustain the inflammatory self-recognition process (Pelfrey et al., 1995; Tanaka et al., 1995; Zhang et al., 1995). Alternatively, regression of autoreactivity may be due to anergy (Correale et al., 1996; DeSilva et al., 1991; Schwartz, 1990; van Parijs et al., 1997) or suppression (Offner et al., 1991; Vandenbark et al., 1989) of the established mature autoreactive repertoire. Experiments designed to determine the relative contributions of deletion, anergy and suppression toward the observed spontaneous regression of self-recognition are currently in progress. The outcome may, one hopes, explain the fundamental mechanism(s) responsible for the inherent instability of the self-recognition process responsible for progression of autoimmune disease.

Acknowledgment. This research was supported by grants NS36054 and NS37476 from the National Institutes of Health USA and by grant RG3070 from the National Multiple Sclerosis Society USA.

REFERENCES

Allen M., Sandberg-Wollheim M., Sjogren K., Erlich H. A., Petterson U. and Gyllensten U. (1994): Association of susceptibility to multiple sclerosis in Sweden with HLA class II DRB1 and DQB1 alleles. Hum. Immunol., **39**, 41–48.

Beck R. W., Cleary P. A., Trobe J. D., Kaufman D. I., Kupersmith M. J., Paty D. W. and Brown C. H. (1993): The effect of corticosteroid for acute optic neuritis on the subsequent development of multiple sclerosis. N. Engl. J. Med., **329**, 1764–1769.

Bhardwaj V., Kumar V., Grewal I. S., Dao T., Lehmann P. V., Geysen H. M. and Sercarz E. E. (1994): T cell determinant structure of myelin basic protein in B10. PL, SJL/J, and their F_1s. J. Immunol., **152**, 3711–3719.

Correale J., Gilmore W., Lopez J., Li S. Q., McMillan M. and Weiner L. P. (1996): Defective post-thymic tolerance mechanisms during the chronic progressive stage of multiple sclerosis. Nat. Med., **2**, 1354–1360.

Cross A. H., Tuohy V. K. and Raine C. S. (1993): Development of reactivity to new myelin antigens during chronic relapsing autoimmune demyelination. Cell. Immunol., **146**, 261–269.

De Silva D. R., Urdahl K. B. and Jenkins M. K. (1991): Clonal anergy is induced *in vitro* by T cell receptor occupancy in the absence of proliferation. J. Immunol., **147**, 3261–3267.

Filippi M., Horsfield M. A., Morrissey S. P., MacManus D. G., Rudge P., McDonald W. I. and Miller D. H. (1994): Quantitative brain MRI lesion load predicts the course of clinically isolated syndromes suggestive of multiple sclerosis. Neurology, **44**, 635–641.

Francis D. A., Thompson A. J., Brookes P., Davey N., Lechler R. I., McDonald W. I. and Batchelor J. R. (1991): Multiple sclerosis and HLA: Is the susceptibility gene really HLA-DR or -DQ? Hum. Immunol., **32**, 119–124.

Gallimore A., Glithero A., Godkin A., Tissot A. C., Pluckthun A., Elliott T., Hengartner H. and Zinkernagel R. (1998): Induction and exhaustion of lymphocytic choriomeningitis virus-specific cytotoxic T lymphocytes visualized using soluble tetrameric major histocompatibility complex class I-peptide complexes. J. Exp. Med., **187**, 1383–1393.

Lehmann P. V., Forsthuber T., Miller A. and Sercarz E. E. (1992): Spreading of T cell autoimmunity to cryptic determinants of an autoantigen. Nature, **358**, 155–157.

Martin R., McFarland H. F. and McFarlin D. E. (1992): Immunological aspects of demyelinating diseases. Annu. Rev. Immunol., **10**, 153–187.

McCarron R. M., Fallis R. J. and McFarlin D. E. (1990): Alterations in T cell antigen specificity and class II restriction during the course of chronic relapsing experimental allergic encephalomyelitis. J. Neuroimmunol., **29**, 73–79.

McRae B. L., Vanderlugt C. L., Dal Canto M. C. and Miller S. D. (1995): Functional evidence for epitope spreading in the relapsing pathology of experimental autoimmune encephalomyelitis. J. Exp. Med., **182**, 75–86.

Mor F. and Coher I. R. (1993): Shifts in the epitopes of myelin basic protein recognized by Lewis rat T cells before, during, and after the induction of experimental autoimmune encephalomyelitis. J. Clin. Invest., **92**, 2199–2206.

Morrissey S. P., Miller D. H., Kendall B. E., Kingsley D. P., Kelly M. A., Francis D. A., MacManus D. G. and Mc Donald W. I. (1993): The significance of brain magnetic resonance imaging abnormalities at presentation with clinically isolated syndromes suggestive of multiple sclerosis. Brain, **116**, 135–146.

Offner H., Hashim G. A. and Vandenbark A. A. (1991): T cell receptor peptide therapy triggers autoregulation of experimental encephalomyelitis. Science, **251**, 430–432.

Pelfrey C. M., Tranquill L. R., Boehme S. A., McFarland H. F. and Lenardo M. J. (1995): Two mechanisms of antigen-specific apoptosis of myelin basic protein (MBP)-specific T lymphocytes derived from multiple sclerosis patients and normal individuals. J. Immunol., **154**, 6191–6202.

Perry L. L., Barzaga-Gilbert E. and Trotter J. L. (1991): T cell sensitization to proteolipid protein in myelin basic protein-induced relapsing experimental allergic encephalomyelitis. J. Neuroimmunol., **33**, 7–15.

Raine C. S. (1984): Biology of disease. Analysis of autoimmune demyelination: its impact upon multiple sclerosis. Lab. Invest., **50**, 608–635.

Schwartz R. H. (1990): A cell culture model for T lymphocyte clonal anergy. Science, **248**, 1349–1356.

Sobel R. A., Tuohy V. K. and Lees M. B. (1991): Parental MHC molecule haplotype expression in (SJL/JxSWR) F_1 mice with acute experimental allergic encephalomyelitis induced with two different synthetic peptides of myelin proteolipid protein. J. Immunol., **146**, 543–549.

Steinman L. (1996): Multiple sclerosis: A coordinated immunological attack against myelin in the central nervous system. Cell, **85**, 299–302.

Tanaka H., Ota K., Ikusaka M., Ejima M. and Maruyama S. (1995): Expression of Fas-antigen on T cells in multiple sclerosis (Japanese). Rinsho Shinkeigaku, **35**, 299–301.

Tuohy V. K., Fritz R. B. and Ben-Nun A. (1994): Self-determinants in autoimmune demyelinating disease: Changes in T-cell response specificity. Curr. Opin. Immunol., **6**, 887–891.

Tuohy V. K. and Thomas D. M. (1995): Sequence 104-117 of myelin proteolipid protein is a cryptic encephalitogenic T cell determinant for SJL/J mice. J. Neuroimmunol., **56**, 161–170.

Tuohy V. K., Yu M., Weinstock-Guttman B. and Kinkel R. P. (1997): Diversity and plasticity of self-recognition during the development of multiple sclerosis. J. Clin. Invest., **99**, 1682–1690.

Tuohy V. K., Yu M., Yin L., Kawczak J. A. and Kinkel R. P. (1999a): Regression and spreading of self-recognition during the development of autoimmune demyelinating disease. J. Autoimmun., **13**, 11–20.

Tuohy V. K., Yu M., Yin L., Kawczak J. A. and Kinkel R. P. (1999b): Spontaneous regression of primary autoreactivity during chronic progression of experimental autoimmune encephalomyelitis and multiple sclerosis. J. Exp. Med., **189**, 1033–1042.

Vandenbark A. A., Hashim G. and Offner H. (1989): Immunization with a synthetic T-cell receptor V-region peptide protects against experimental autoimmune encephalomyelitis. Nature, **341**, 541–544.

Vanderlugt C. J. and Miller S. D. (1996): Epitope spreading. Curr. Opin. Immunol., **8**, 831–836.

Van Parijs L. V., Perez V. L., Biuckians A., Maki R. G., London C. A. and Abbas A. K. (1997): Role of interleukin 12 and costimulators in T cell anergy *in vivo*. J. Exp. Med., **186**, 1119–1128.

Yu M., Johnson J. M. and Tuohy V. K. (1996a): A predictable sequential determinant spreading cascade invariably accompanies progression of experimental autoimmune encephalomyelitis: A basis for peptide-specific therapy after onset of clinical disease. J. Exp. Med., **183**, 1777–1788.

Yu M., Johnson J. M. and Tuohy V. K. (1996b): Generation of autonomously pathogenic neoautoreactive Th1 cells during the development of the determinant spreading cascade in murine autoimmune encephalomyelitis. J. Neurosci. Res., **45**, 463–470.

Yu M., Kinkel R. P., Weinstock-Guttman B., Cook D. J. and Tuohy V. K. (1998): HLA-DP: A class II restriction molecule involved in epitope spreading during the development of multiple sclerosis. Hum. Immunol., **59**, 15–24.

Zhang J., Vandevyver C., Stinissen P. and Raus J. (1995): *In vivo* clonotypic regulation of human myelin basic protein-reactive T cells by T cell vaccination. J. Immunol., **155**, 5868–5877.

A ROLE FOR NF-κB AND THE PROTEASOME IN AUTOIMMUNITY

TAKUMA HAYASHI and DENISE FAUSTMAN

Immunobiology Laboratory, Massachusetts General Hospital, and Harvard Medical School, Charlestown, MA 02129, USA

Abstract Type 1 diabetes (also known as insulin-dependent diabetes mellitus or juvenile--onset diabetes) is usually caused by T cell-mediated autoimmunity, with a prediabetic state characterized by the production of autoantibodies specific for proteins expressed by pancreatic β cells. The non-obese diabetic (NOD) mouse is a spontaneous model of type 1 diabetes with a strong genetic component that maps to the major histocompatibility complex (MHC) region of the genome. A specific proteasome defect has been identified in NOD mouse lymphocytes that results from down-regulation of expression of the proteasome subunit LMP2, which is encoded by a gene in the MHC genomic region. This defect both prevents the proteolytic processing required for the production and activation of the transcription factor nuclear factor κB (NF-κB), which plays important roles in immune and inflammatory responses, as well as increases the susceptibility of the affected cells to apoptosis induced by tumor necrosis factor α (TNF-α). The proteasome dysfunction is both tissue and developmental stage specific and likely contributes to disease pathogenesis and tissue targeting.

Key words: type 1 diabetes; proteasome; LMP2; apoptosis; non-obese diabetic mouse; NF-κB.

Abbreviations used: MHC – major histocompatibility complex, NOD – non-obese diabetic, NF-κB – nuclear factor κB, IL – interleukin, TNF-α – tumor necrosis factor α, IKK – IκB kinase, EMSA – electrophoretic mobility-shift assay, NIK – NF--κB-inducing kinase, E – embryonic day, GM-CSF – granulocyte-macrophage colony-stimulating factor.

1. GENETIC RISK FACTORS FOR TYPE 1 DIABETES LOCATED IN THE MHC REGION OF THE GENOME

Type 1 diabetes mellitus is an autoimmune disease with genetic risk factors that map to the MHC region of the genome. In both human type 1 diabetes and two rodent models (NOD mouse and BB rat) of the disease, pan-

A. Górski et al. (eds.), Autoimmunity, 49–71.

creatic β cells are selectively destroyed by a chronic autoimmune reaction (Crisa et al., 1992; Rabinovitch and Skyler, 1998). The NOD mouse model of diabetes is characterized by a marked gender difference with regard to the incidence of disease. In females, the onset of diabetes occurs at ~20 to 40 weeks of age and the number of animals that develop overt diabetes increases with age, with the cumulative incidence of the disease reaching 85% by 40 weeks of age. In contrast, in male mice, although the onset of diabetes is also first apparent at ~20 weeks of age, only ~10 to 30% of animals are affected by the age of 40 weeks (Makino et al., 1980).

The MHC region of the genome contains immune response genes that are important in T cell education and in antigen presentation by both MHC class I and class II molecules. Studies of both humans and rodents have implicated the centrally located MHC class II genes as a major statistical risk factor for autoimmune disease. A clear functional derangement in MHC class II genes has been less clear. In contrast, cellular derangements in maturation markers or antigen presentation functions are commonly observed in NOD and diabetic humans and can be depicted by decreased expression of cell maturation antigens such as CD45 or altered levels of conformationally correct MHC class I and self-peptide complexes (Faustman et al., 1989; Faustman et al., 1991a; 1991b; Jansen et al., 1995; Smerdon et al., 1993). Evidence based on functional assays suggests human autoimmune diseases may be associated with impairment of protein processing controlled by the MHC. Thus, cytosolic extracts of lymphocytes from humans with type 1 diabetes or NOD mice exhibit altered patterns of cleavage of test substrates by the proteasome, resulting in the generation of peptides that are poorly suited to assembly with MHC class I molecules (Fu et al., 1998; Hayashi and Faustman, 1999). Furthermore, individuals with diverse autoimmune diseases, including type 1 diabetes, multiple sclerosis and rheumatoid arthritis, exhibit decreased expression of peptide-loaded MHC class I molecules on the surface of their lymphocytes (Faustman et al., 1991a; Fu et al., 1993; Li et al., 1995). Moreover, clinical studies have shown that the antigen-presentation defect correlates with disease expression in identical twins with type 1 diabetes (Faustman et al., 1991a). The genes responsible for these peptide-processing defects associated with human autoimmune diseases map to the MHC region of the genome (Fu et al., 1998), suggesting that a similar MHC-region abnormality might underlie these various conditions.

The MHC in humans and rodents contains many candidate genes, including those encoding the TAP peptide transporters and LMP proteasome subunits, that, when malfunctioning, might be responsible for impaired assembly of peptide-loaded MHC class I molecules. Thus, for example, both LMP2 and LMP7 are encoded by genes located in the MHC region of the genome;

these proteins are constitutively expressed in most cell types, but their expression is markedly increased in antigen-presenting cells or lymphoid cells by interferon γ treatment (Fruh et al., 1992; Griffin et al., 1998; Hisamatsu et al., 1996; Van Kaer et al., 1994). Furthermore, these genes, since their discovery, have been strong candidates for high risk of developing type 1 diabetes, not only because of their chromosomal location, but also due to the fact that transgenic mice with ablation of these genes have abnormal T cell selection and autoreactivity against transplants of syngeneic normal tissues (Aldrich et al., 1994; Faustman et al., 1991a; Glas et al., 1994; Van Kaer et al., 1994; Wakatsuki et al., 1994).

Ubiquitin-dependent proteolysis by the proteasome plays an essential role in various important cellular processes, including cell cycle progression, gene transcription and signal transduction (Coux et al., 1998; Goldberg, 1995). In many instances, the target protein is marked for degradation or processing by both phosphorylation and ubiquitination. Cleavage of endogenous proteins by the proteasome also generates small self-peptide fragments that contribute to T cell education after presentation by MHC class I molecules. Although, in general, the proteasome exhibits minimal variability in substrate selectivity and subunit composition, incorporation of the LMP2 and LMP7 subunits during assembly of the proteasome changes its specificity for self-proteins in such a manner that the suitability of the generated peptides for presentation in the peptide-binding groove of MHC class I molecules is increased (Belich et al., 1994; Gaczynska et al., 1996). Expression of the LMP2 gene is down-regulated in lymphocytes derived from NOD mice (Yan et al., 1997), thereby explaining the altered T cell education towards self.

2. ACTIVATION OF NF-κB BY THE PROTEASOME PROCESSING PATHWAY

The proteasome also plays an important role in the processing and activation of the NF-κB/Rel superfamily and other members of the Rel family of transcription factors, which are sequestered in the cytoplasm as a result of their association with the IκB family (Baldwin, 1996) (Fig. 1). Until recently it was thought that the entire proteasome structure and all of its contained subunits were required for NF-κB activation. Additionally inducible MHC-linked proteasome units, LMP2 and LMP7, were obligatory for MHC class I display, although these were expressed constitutively as well. The highly inducible LMP2 and LMP7 subunits were known to be only obligatory for the processing of other protein substrates.

NF-κB is activated in response to various extracellular stimuli, including interleukin 1 (IL-1), lipopolysaccharide and tumor necrosis factor α (TNF-α) (Baeuerle and Baltimore, 1996; Baldwin, 1996; Thanos and Maniatis, 1995; Verma et al., 1995) (Fig. 1). Activated NF-κB, in turn, has been implicated in the regulation of gene transcription that contributes to cytokine generation, expression of cell surface adhesion epitopes, lymphocyte maturation, protection from TNF-α-induced apoptosis, and antigen processing and presentation by MHC class I molecules (Beg and Baltimore, 1996; Bohnline et al., 1988; Cross et al., 1989; Tan et al., 1992; Van Antwerp et al., 1996). Insights into the various biological functions of NF-κB have been obtained by the gener-

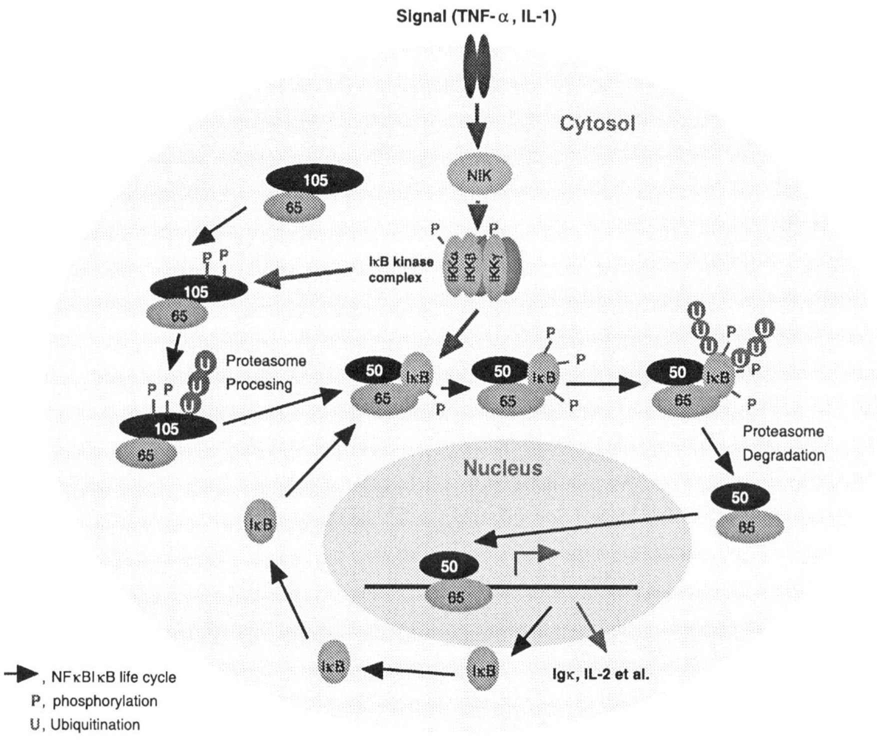

Figure 1. Schematic representation of the molecular mechanism of NF-κB activation. Extracellular signals such as TNF-α and IL-1 trigger the activation of NF-κB-inducing kinase (NIK), which, in turn, phosphorylates the IκB kinase (IKK) complex. Association of the p105-p65 heterodimer with the IKK complex results in the phosphorylation of p105, which is followed by its ubiquitination and processing by the proteasome. The resulting p50-p65 complex then associates with IκBα. Association of the p50-p65-IκBα complex with the IKK complex results in the phosphorylation of IκBα and its subsequent ubiquitination and degradation by the proteasome. The released p50-p65 heterodimer translocates to the nucleus, where it activates the transcription of target genes, including those encoding IκBα, IL-2, and the immunoglobulin κ chain (Igκ)

ation of knockout mice lacking either subunits of this protein or associated regulatory proteins (Burkly et al., 1995; Bushdid et al., 1998; Caamano et al., 1998; Franzoso et al., 1997; Hu et al., 1999; Kanegae et al., 1998; Kontgen et al., 1995; Li et al., 1999a; 1999b; Takeda et al., 1999; Weih et al., 1995).

Active NF-κB exists predominantly as a heterodimer composed of p65 (RelA) and either p50 or p52 subunits. The p50 and p52 subunits are generated constitutively but significantly augmented by certain stimuli such as IL-1 and TNF-α. The proteasome-mediated removal of the carboxyl termini of p105 and p100 precursors, respectively (Coux and Goldberg, 1998; Fan and Maniatis, 1991; Lin et al., 1998; Palombella et al., 1994; Schmid et al., 1991; Sears et al., 1998), and this proteasome cleavage is obligatory for the active p65-p50 subunit (Fig. 1). In the cytoplasm of resting cells, NF-κB is associated with the inhibitory protein IκBα (Ghosh and Baltimore, 1990; Hayashi et al., 1993a; 1993b). Cell stimulation results in the phosphorylation of IκBα by the IκB kinase (IKK) complex and its degradation by the ubiquitin-proteasome pathway, thereby allowing the p50-p65 or p52-p65 heterodimer to translocate to the nucleus and initiate the transcription of target genes (Belich et al., 1999; Ghosh and Baltimore, 1990; MacKichan et al., 1996; Neri et al., 1991; Palombella et al., 1994) (Fig. 1). Complexes of p65 with p105 have also been detected, but these do not appear to translocate rapidly to the nucleus in response to cell stimulation (Lin et al., 1970; Sun et al., 1994).

3. IMPAIRED EXPRESSION AND ACTIVITY OF NF-κB IN NOD MOUSE LYMPHOCYTES

The role of the proteasome in the processing and activation of NF-κB is established but only recently has this been linked to LMP2 subunit expression (Hayashi and Faustman, 1999). The reduced *Lmp2* gene expression in lymphocytes from NOD (Yan et al., 1997) prompted us to examine the effect of TNF-α on the activation of NF-κB in spleen cells derived from BALB/c and NOD mice. Incubation of human T cell lymphoma Molt-4 cells or BALB/c mouse spleen cells, as controls, with TNF-α (10 ng/ml) for 4 h resulted in a marked increase in the DNA-binding activity of NF-κB in the nucleus, as determined by electrophoretic mobility-shift assay (Fig. 2A). In contrast, TNF-α had little effect on NF-κB activity in the nucleus of spleen cells from NOD mice (male or female). The DNA-binding activity of NF-κB in detergent-treated cytosolic extracts of NOD mouse spleen cells was also markedly reduced compared with that observed in such extracts of Molt-4 or BALB/c mouse spleen cells (Fig. 2A). The DNA-binding activities of the transcription factors SP1 and AP1 did not differ between nuclear extracts of

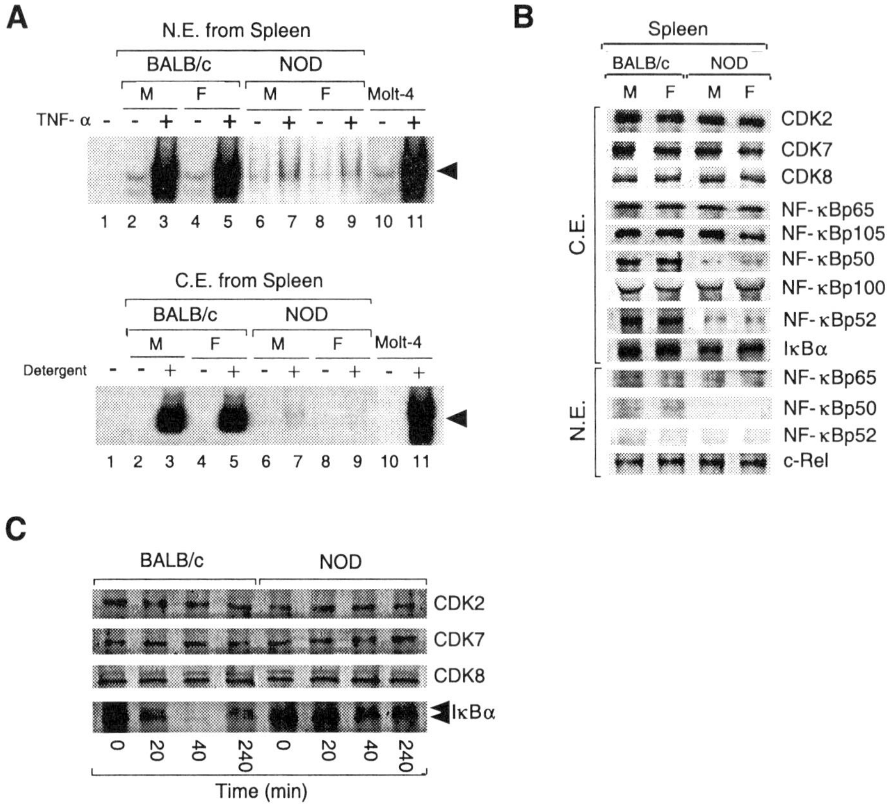

Figure 2. Impaired expression and activation of NF-κB in NOD mouse splenocytes. A – upper panel: the DNA-binding activity of NF-κB in nuclear extracts (N. E.) prepared from NOD and BALB/c mouse (M – male; F – female) splenocytes, as well as from Molt-4 cells, after incubation of cells in the absence (–) or presence (+) of TNF-α (10 ng/ml) for 4 h. Lane 1 corresponds to a negative control in which no nuclear extract was added to the reaction mixture. The arrowhead indicates the specific DNA-protein complex. Lower panel: similarly the DNA-binding activity of NF-κB in cytosolic extracts (C. E.) of BALB/c and NOD mouse lymphocytes and of Molt-4 cells after incubation of cytosolic extracts in the absence (–) or presence (+) of detergent (NP-40 and deoxycholate). B – immunoblot analysis of NF--κB subunits (p65, p52, p50) and their precursors (p105, p100), c-Rel, IκBα, and cyclin-dependent kinases (CDKs) in cytosolic and nuclear extracts of unstimulated spleen cells from BALB/c and NOD mice. C – effect of TNF-α on the abundance of IκBα in spleen cells of BALB/c and NOD female mice. Splenocytes were incubated with TNF-α (10 ng/ml) for the indicated times, after which cytosolic extracts were prepared and subjected to immunoblot analysis with antibodies to IκBα or to CDKs. Arrowheads indicate phosphorylated (upper band) and nonphosphorylated (lower band) forms of IκBα. Reproduced with permission from reference (Hayashi and Faustman, 1999)

BALB/c and NOD mouse spleen cells, indicating that the NF-κB defect in the NOD mouse spleen cells was specific.

The basal expression of NF-κB subunits in cytosolic and nuclear extracts of BALB/c and NOD splenocytes was also examined by immunoblot analysis (Fig. 2B). The amounts of p65, the p50 precursor p105, and the p52 precursor p100, as well as those of IκBα and the cyclin-dependent kinases CDK8, CDK7, and CDK2 (assayed as internal controls), in cytosolic extracts, did not differ markedly between BALB/c and NOD mouse cells. However, the abundance of p50 and p52 in the cytosolic extracts prepared from NOD splenocytes (male and female) was markedly reduced relative to that in splenocytes from BALB/c mice. Similarly, whereas the amounts of p65 and c-Rel were similar in nuclear extracts of splenocytes from the two mouse strains, the amounts of p50 and p52 were reduced in the nuclear extracts from NOD mice.

We also investigated the effects of TNF-α on the abundance of IκBα in splenocytes from BALB/c and NOD mice (Fig. 2C). Exposure of BALB/c cells to TNF-α for 40 min resulted in the almost complete disappearance of IκBα from the cytosol, although this protein began to reappear by 240 min. In contrast, the amount of IκBα in the cytosol of NOD mouse spleen cells was not markedly affected by exposure of the cells to TNF-α for up to 240 min. The phosphorylated form of IκBα was detected as the upper of two immunoreactive bands in cytosolic extracts of TNF-α-treated spleen cells from both BALB/c and NOD mice. The basal expression of NF-κB-inducing kinase (NIK), which is required for the TNF-α-induced phosphorylation, was similar in cytosolic extracts of spleen cells from both BALB/c and NOD mice. These various results thus suggested that the proteasomal processing of the NF-κB subunit precursors p105 and p100 as well as the proteasome-mediated degradation of IκBα were impaired in NOD mouse lymphocytes.

4. IMPAIRED PROTEASOMAL PROCESSING OF P105 TO P50 BY NOD MOUSE LYMPHOCYTE EXTRACTS

We next investigated whether the reduced expression of p50 in NOD mouse lymphocytes might be attributable to a defect in p50 generation by the ATP-dependent ubiquitin-proteasome pathway with the use of an *in vitro* processing assay (Fan and Maniatis, 1991; Palombella et al., 1994). Whereas incubation of recombinant p105 with cytosolic extracts of BALB/c splenocytes in the presence of ATP resulted in the generation of substantial amounts of p50 (Fig. 3A), little such conversion of p105 to p50 was apparent in incubations performed with extracts of NOD mouse cells; moreover, this defect appeared more pronounced for NOD females than for NOD males. To confirm that the formation of p50 in this *in vitro* processing assay was mediated by the ubiquitin-proteasome pathway, we examined the effect of MG115. This compound is a potent inhibitor of the chymotryptic site on the 20S proteasome particle and inhibits the degradation of ubiquitin-conjugated proteins in cell extracts; at a concentration of 50 μM, it was previously shown to prevent the generation of p50 from p105 (Palombella et al., 1994). We also found that the processing of p105 by mouse splenocyte extracts was completely inhibited by MG115 at a concentration of 50 μM (Fig. 3A).

Phosphorylation of a PEST-rich domain downstream of the ankyrin repeats of p105 is induced by exposure of cells to TNF-α (Belich et al., 1999; MacKichan et al., 1996; Naumann and Scheidereit, 1994). We therefore examined the phosphorylation status of recombinant p105 after incubation with [γ-^{32}P] ATP and cytosolic extracts of splenocytes from BALB/c and NOD mice. The p105 protein was phosphorylated to similar extents on incubation with extracts from the two strains of mice, indicating that the activity of the responsible kinase (IKK) is normal in NOD mouse spleen cells. Ubiquitination of the ankyrin repeats of p105 is also thought to be required for the proteolytic processing of this protein (Orian et al., 1995; Pahl and Baeuerle, 1996; Palombella et al., 1994). We therefore measured the ubiquitination of recombinant p105 after incubation with cytosolic extracts of BALB/c and NOD mouse splenocytes. Cross-linking of ubiquitin-p105 complexes with glutaraldehyde, followed by the immunoprecipitation of these complexes with antibodies to p50 and immunoblot analysis with antibodies to ubiquitin, revealed no differences between the time courses of p105 ubiquitination catalyzed by the extracts from BALB/c and NOD mice (Hayashi and Faustman, 1999). Together, these observations suggested that the defect in p50 expression in NOD mouse lymphocytes was localized at the level of proteasomal processing of p105.

5. DEFICIENCY OF THE PROTEASOMAL SUBUNIT LMP2 IN NOD MOUSE SPLEEN CELLS

The 26S proteasome comprises 20S and 19S components (Fig. 3C). On the basis of sequence similarity, all 20S proteasomal subunits can be classified into one of two groups, α and β, with the members of the two groups exhibiting distinct structural and functional roles. The seven α subunits and the seven β subunits form the outer and inner rings, respectively, that constitute the 20S proteasome, and each subunit is located in a specific position within these rings (Fig. 3C).

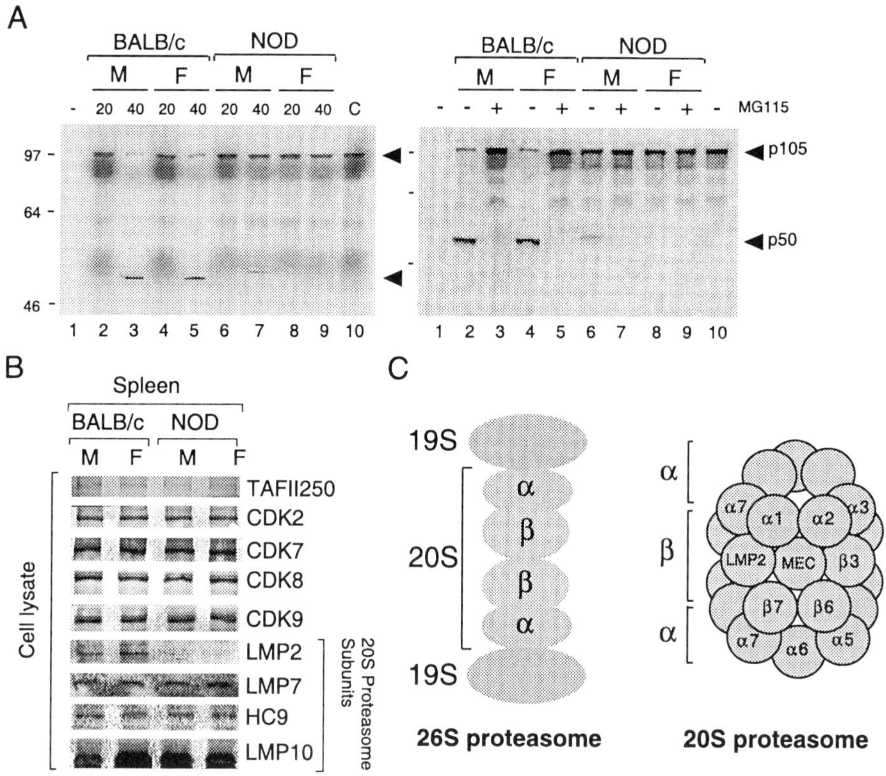

Figure 3. Impaired proteasomal processing of p105 by and expression of LMP2 in extracts of NOD mouse spenocytes. A – purified recombinant ^{35}S-labeled p105 was incubated for 90 min at 30°C in the presence of 10 mM ATP and cytosolic extracts of male or female BALB/c or NOD mouse splenocytes (20 or 40 μg of protein in left panel; 40 μg of protein in right panel). For the right panel, incubations were also performed in the absence (–) or presence (+) of 50 μM MG115. Lanes 1 correspond to reaction mixtures without substrate, and lanes 10 correspond to reaction mixtures without added cytosolic extract. The reaction mixtures were analyzed by SDS-polyacrylamide gel electrophoresis and autoradiography. The positions of molecular size standards (shown in kilodaltons) are indicated on the left. B – the cell lysates of spleen cells from male and female BALB/c and NOD mice were subjected to immunoblot analysis with antibodies specific for the indicated 20S proteasome subunits or, as controls, with antibodies to various CDKs or to TAFII250. C – schematic representations of 26S and 20S proteasomes. Panels A and B are reproduced with permission from reference (Hayashi and Faustman, 1999)

Immunoblot analysis revealed the presence of the LMP2 proteasome subunit in cytosolic extracts of BALB/c splenocytes but not in those of NOD mouse splenocytes (Fig. 3B). Basal expression of the proteasome subunits LMP7, LMP10 and HC9 did not differ between BALB/c and NOD mice. Immunoblot analysis of lysates of fibroblasts derived from 13.5-day BALB/c and NOD mouse embryos revealed no differences in the amounts of LMP2, LMP7, LMP10 and HC9 or in those of NF-κB subunits (p65, p52, p50) and precursors (p105, p100) between the two strains (Hayashi and Faustman, unpublished data). The tissue specificity of the defect in LMP2 expression was also evaluated by examining the abundance of this protein in freshly isolated pancreatic islets of Langerhans from BALB/c and NOD mice. Islet extracts from the two mouse strains contained similar amounts of LMP2 (Hayashi and Faustman, unpublished data). The proteasome defect in NOD mice thus appears restricted to the lymphoid lineage. We also examined the ability of cytosolic extracts of lymphocytes from LMP2 knockout mice to process recombinant p105 to p50 (Hayashi and Faustman, 1999; 2000). Similar to the cytosolic extracts of NOD mouse splenocytes, those of the LMP2 knockout mice failed to catalyze p105 processing to p50 in the presence of ATP (Hayashi and Faustman, 1999; 2000).

6. INCREASED SENSITIVITY OF NOD MOUSE LYMPHOCYTES TO TNF-α-INDUCED APOPTOSIS

Evidence indicates that NF-κB is an important protector from apoptosis (Cui et al., 1997). The hepatic apoptosis observed in embryos of p65 or IKKβ knockout mice appears to result from the associated defects in NF-κB activation (Beg and Baltimore, 1996; Beg et al., 1995; Horwitz et al., 1997; Li et al., 1999a; Tanaka et al., 1999). The activation of NF-κB by the ubiquitin-proteasome pathway is thought to protect cells from TNF-α-induced cell death (Beg and Baltimore, 1996; Van Antwerp et al., 1996; Wang et al., 1996; Wu et al., 1996) (Fig. 4). Thus, inhibition of the nuclear translocation of NF-κB enhances the apoptotic effect of TNF-α. The anti-apoptotic effect of NF-κB is likely mediated by the activation of genes that encode survival proteins (Fig. 4).

We investigated the effect of TNF-α on the viability of NOD mouse lymphocytes, in which TNF-α-induced activation of NF-κB is impaired. Whereas incubation of BALB/c splenocytes with various concentrations (2 to 20 ng/ml) of TNF-α for 24 h had virtually no effect on cell survival, TNF-α induced a dose-dependent decrease in the survival of splenocytes derived from male or female NOD mice (Hayashi and Faustman, 1999). Similarly, whereas incubation of BALB/c splenocytes with TNF-α at 10 ng/ml for up to 48 h had no effect on cell viability, the survival of NOD splenocytes was already markedly reduced after incubation with the same concentration of TNF-α for only 12 h (Hayashi and Faustman, 1999). The toxic effect of TNF-α on NOD mouse lymphocytes also appeared more pronounced for

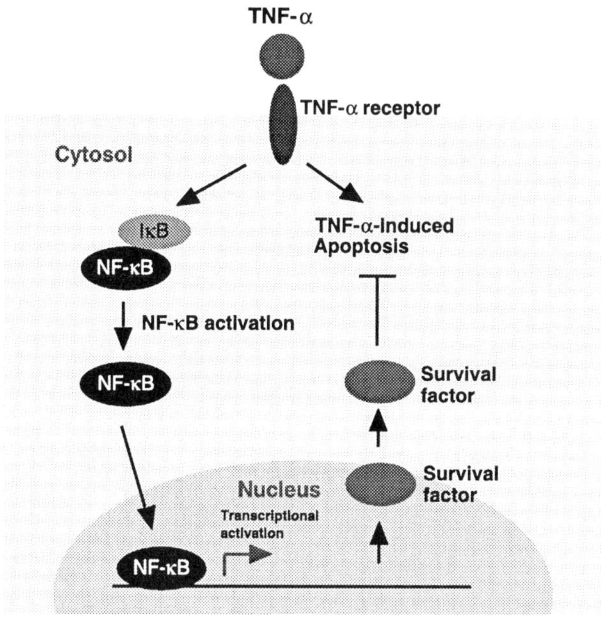

Figure 4. Proposed mechanism for the inhibition by NF-κB of TNF-α-induced apoptosis. The pro-apoptotic effect of TNF-α is thought to be counteracted by the simultaneous activation of NF-κB, which exerts its anti-apoptotic effect by activating the transcription of target genes that encode cell survival-promoting proteins

female than for male animals. Exposure of lymphocytes from LMP2 knockout mice to TNF-α also resulted in marked cell death (Hayashi and Faustman, 1999). Analysis of DNA fragmentation by agarose gel electrophoresis confirmed that TNF-α-induced a pattern of internucleosomal fragmentation characteristic of apoptosis in lymphocytes from NOD mice and LMP2 knockout mice, whereas it did not induce DNA fragmentation in those from BALB/c mice (Hayashi and Faustman, 1999). Thus, it is likely that the toxicity of TNF-α for NOD mouse lymphocytes is attributable to the proteasome-associated defect in NF-κB activation in these cells.

TNF-α also reduced the viability of spleen cells derived from 7-day-old NOD mice, but to a lesser extent than it did in cells derived from adult animals; the cytokine had no effect on the viability of spleen cells derived from 7-day-old BALB/c mice (Hayashi and Faustman, unpublished data). Whereas TNF-α had no effect on the viability of cultured macrophages derived from 13.5-day BALB/c or NOD mouse fetal liver, it induced a dose- and time-dependent decrease in the viability of such cells derived from the LMP2 knockout mouse fetal liver at the same stage of development (Hayashi and Faustman, 1999). Similarly, TNF-α had no effect on the viability of cultured

BALB/c or NOD mouse embryonic fibroblasts, whereas TNF-α treatment of such cells derived from LMP2 knockout mice resulted in prominent cell death (Hayashi and Faustman, unpublished data). Although disruption of the NF-κB p65 or IKKβ genes is associated with marked abnormalities in liver development (Beg and Baltimore, 1996; Beg et al., 1995; Li et al., 1999a; Tanaka et al., 1999), hematoxylin-eosin staining of liver sections from 6-week--old NOD mice did not reveal any apparent liver defects (Hayashi and Faustman, 1999).

7. IMPAIRED GRANULOCYTE-MACROPHAGE COLONY FORMATION BY NOD MOUSE SPLEEN CELLS

NF-κB also plays an important role in the maturation of lymphocytes and monocytes. We therefore examined the development of the granulocyte-macrophage cell lineage in splenocytes isolated from 6-week-old NOD and BALB/c mice. Colony-formation assays revealed that, whereas granulocyte--macrophage colony-stimulating factor (GM-CSF) induced the formation of clusters of mature granulocytes-macrophages in BALB/c mouse splenocytes, the formation of such clusters was impaired in splenocytes from NOD mice (Fig. 5, A through D). Furthermore, whereas exposure of GM-CSF-treated spleen cell cultures from BALB/c mice to TNF-α had no effect on cell viability or colony development, TNF-α induced the death of all cells in the NOD mouse cultures (Fig. 5, E through H).

The specificity of the developmental defect and cytotoxic effect of TNF-α in the granulocyte-macrophage lineage of NOD mice was investigated by examining colony-forming units of erythrocytes in cultures of spleen cells derived from 6-week-old BALB/c and NOD animals. Erythrocyte colony formation appeared normal in erythropoietin-supplemented cultures of NOD mouse spleen cells, compared to that observed in spleen cells from BALB/c mice (Hayashi and Faustman, 1999). Moreover, TNF-α had no effect on erythrocyte colony formation, which is known to require NF-κB, in spleen cells from either BALB/c or NOD mice. These results suggest that a lack of

Figure 5. Impaired granulocyte-macrophage colony formation and increased sensitivity to TNF-α-induced apoptosis in NOD mouse spleen cells. Spleen cells (1×10^5) derived from 6--week-old male or female BALB/c and NOD mice were mixed with 1.3% methylcellulose dissolved in culture medium and layered onto a bed of 0.53% agarose in culture medium. Cells were cultured for 3 weeks in the presence of GM-CSF (20 ng/ml) and in the absence or presence of TNF-α (20 ng/ml), as indicated

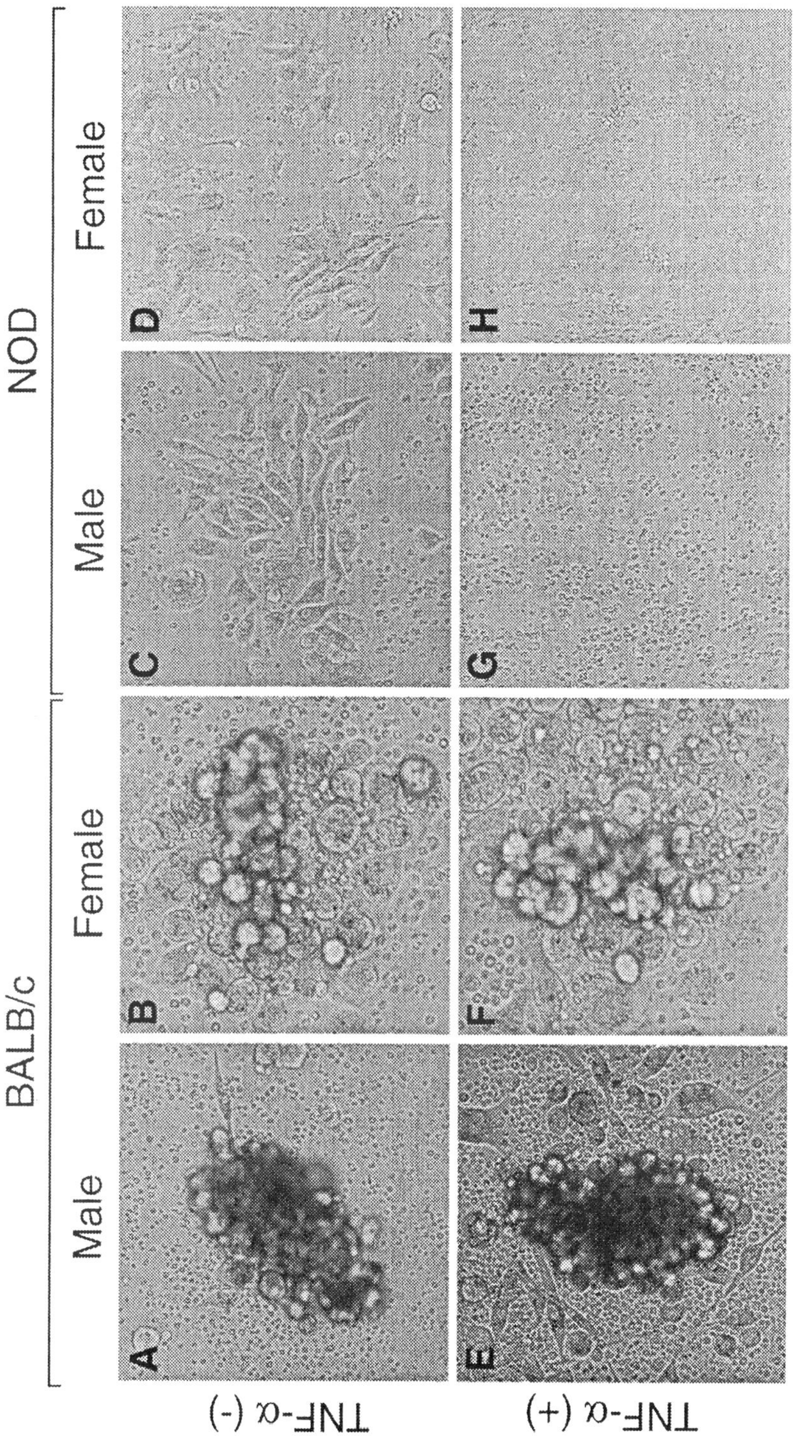
BALB/c
NOD
Male
Female
Male
Female
A
B
C
D
E
F
G
H
TNF-α (-)
TNF-α (+)

NF-κB activation in granulocyte-macrophage precursors derived from NOD mice at 6 weeks of age impairs the maturation of these cells and renders them susceptible to the cytotoxic effect of TNF-α. In contrast, NF-κB appears to be functional in the erythrocyte lineage of these mice, which appears to develop normally and to be resistant to TNF-α-induced apoptosis. Given that TNF-α had no effect on the viability of cultured macrophages derived from the 13.5-day BALB/c or NOD mouse fetal liver, the proteasome defect in these animals appears to be both cell type and developmental stage specific.

8. GENDER/AGE-RELATED AND TISSUE SPECIFIC PROTEASOME DYSFUNCTION AND DISEASE EXPRESSION

The incidence of diabetes is markedly greater in NOD females than in NOD males. Most human autoimmune diseases are also preferentially expressed in females. Consistent with a role for defective proteasome and NF-κB function in NOD mouse diabetes, a recent report has shown that cytosolic extracts of splenocytes from male NOD mice were able to convert a small proportion of recombinant p105 to p50, albeit an aberrantly sized protein fragment (Hayashi and Faustman, 1999). Splenocyte extracts from female animals did not generate any detectable p50 protein in this assay (Hayashi and Faustman, 1999). Furthermore, both the time course and dose--response relation for the effect of TNF-α on cell viability revealed that the sensitivity of splenocytes from NOD females to this cytokine was greater than that of cells from NOD males (Hayashi and Faustman, 1999).

The characteristics of knockout mice that lack Rel family proteins or LMP2 show partial overlap with those of NOD mice (Beg et al., 1995; Burkly et al., 1995; Kontgen et al., 1995; Van Kaer et al., 1994; Weih et al., 1995). However, LMP2-deficient mice do not develop diabetes by 32 weeks of age (Faustman, unpublished observation), consistent with the contribution of multiple chromosomal regions to disease penetrance in both NOD mice and humans. The homogeneous nature of the gene defect in all tissues of LMP2 knockout mice differs from the apparent developmental stage and tissue specificity of the proteasome defect in NOD mice, which might underlie target selection in disease expression. LMP2-deficient and other knockout mice with defects in the assembly of MHC class I molecules with self-peptides destroy transplanted syngeneic tissues from control animals (Freland et al., 1998; Li and Faustman, 1993; Vidal-Puig and Faustman, 1994). Target cell loss might thus result from preferential direct attack by cytotoxic T lymphocytes in the early stages of autoimmune disease.

The marked pro-apoptotic effect of TNF-α in NOD mouse lymphocytes also might indicate a role for this cytokine in early β-cell destruction in these animals. Such a mechanism of β-cell death would require that the β cells exhibit the same proteasome defect as that of NOD mouse lymphocytes, characterized by loss of LMP2 expression, aberrant NF-κB activation, increased sensitivity to the cytotoxic effect of TNF-α and reduced expression of peptide-filled MHC class I molecules on the cell surface. However, one of the early pathological features of autoimmune diabetes in both humans and rodent models is hyperexpression of correctly assembled MHC class I molecules on the surface of β cells (Foulis, 1987; Hanafusa et al., 1990; Kay et al., 1991; Ono et al., 1988; Stephens et al., 1997; Vives-Pi et al., 1996; Weringer and Like, 1988), a phenomenon that requires an intact proteasome function. Studies of both humans and animals with diabetes or other autoimmune diseases suggest that discordance in the regulation of MHC-linked genes between tissues might confer target specificity for attack by cytotoxic T lymphocytes (Fig. 6) (Hayashi and Faustman, 1999).

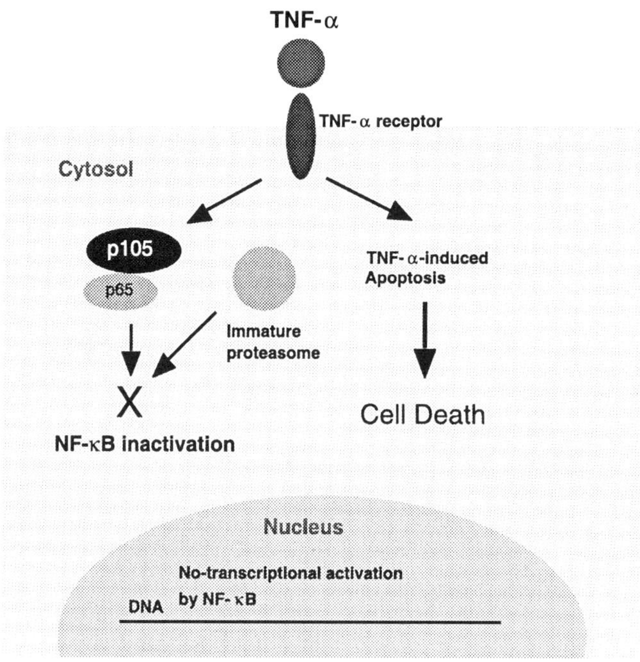

Figure 6. A model for TNF-α-induced apoptosis of NOD lymphocytes. Depicted is a possible mechanism to describe TNF-α-induced apoptosis of NOD lymphocytes. The TNF-α signaling pathway leads to an unknown pro-apoptotic signal. Defective NF-κB activation causes the inactivated expression of genes encoding anti-apoptotic factor, which allow the cell to survive and are not induced, inducing a time- and dose-dependent decrease in cell survival

Macrophages and fibroblasts derived from 13.5-day NOD mouse embryos exhibited normal cell growth and resistance to TNF-α cytotoxicity. In contrast, TNF-α induced a marked pro-apoptotic effect in the corresponding cell types derived from LMP2 knockout mice. TNF-α also induced a relatively small decrease in the viability of spleen cells derived from 7-day-old NOD mice, but had no such effect on corresponding cells from BALB/c mice. In contrast, lymphoid cells of splenic origin, lung macrophages (Kupffer cells) and granulocytes-macrophages from 6–8-week old NOD mice exhibited reduced LMP2 expression, impaired NF-κB activation and increased sensitivity to the cytotoxic effect of TNF-α (Hayashi and Faustman, 1999). Furthermore, consistent with a role for the proteasome and NF-κB in normal cell growth, culture of spleen cells from 6-week-old NOD mice with GM-CSF failed to induce normal expansion of the granulocyte-macrophage cell lineage. The islets of Langerhans, liver, and erythrocytes of 6–8-week-old NOD mice appeared normal. The ability of NOD mouse macrophages to activate regulatory T cells in an autologous mixed lymphocyte reaction has also recently been shown to be impaired (Atkinson and Leiter, 1999).

The age-dependent proteasome defect in the macrophages of NOD mice likely explains some of the important features of disease development in these animals. Thus, NOD mice show no signs of autoimmunity at ages up to 3 weeks. At 5 weeks and older, insulitis begins to appear, and by 8 weeks of age autoantibodies are detectable. The insulitis gradually increases in intensity, with complete destruction of islets usually apparent by 30 weeks of age (Makino et al., 1980). Furthermore, the outcomes of various interventions and treatments in NOD mice are age dependent. For instance, the administration of TNF-α to animals older than 6 weeks has been shown to sometimes prevent the development of diabetes, whereas the same treatment in animals younger than 4 weeks has no effect or a detrimental effect (Yang et al., 1994). Therefore, both the time course of histopathology of autoreactivity and the paradoxical responses to TNF-α treatment parallel the altered developmental regulation of LMP2 expression and NF-κB activity in these animals.

9. DEFECTIVE PROTEASOME FUNCTION AND AUTOIMMUNITY

The ubiquitin-proteasome pathway plays an essential role in many important biological processes (Maniatis, 1999). Protein degradation by this pathway thus generates peptides for presentation by MHC class I molecules and either activates or inactivates transcription factors. In general, the proteasome subunits vary minimally among eukaryotic cells. However, the interferon γ-induced expression of the MHC-encoded proteasome subunits LMP2 and LMP7 is thought to promote the generation of endogenous peptides compatible with the peptide-binding cleft of MHC class I molecules (Akiyama et al., 1994; Belich et al., 1994). The MHC-encoded proteasome subunits also play a role in general proteasome function, including the processing and activation of NF-κB.

The defect in proteasome function in NOD mouse splenocytes is attributable to a loss of expression of the LMP2 subunit and was evident from the impaired proteolytic processing of the p105 precursor of the NF-κB subunit p50 *in vitro* as well as from the lack of degradation of phosphorylated IκBα in these cells in response to TNF-α. This defect confers sensitivity on the affected cells to the cytotoxic effect of TNF-α. The role of LMP2 in NF-κB activation was confirmed by the observations that cytosolic extracts of lymphocytes from LMP2 knockout mice also failed to convert p105 to p50 and that only NOD mouse tissues that lack LMP2 protein showed impaired activation of NF-κB and sensitivity to TNF-α-induced apoptosis (Hayashi and Faustman, 1999; 2000). Our data indicate that the defect in LMP2 protein production in NOD mice is both developmental stage (age) and tissue specific. Thus, NOD macrophages and fibroblasts from 13.5-day embryos showed normal levels of LMP2 expression and were resistant to the cytotoxic effect of TNF-α. In contrast, splenocytes, granulocytes-macrophages and lung Kupffer cells from 6–8-week-old NOD mice lack LMP2 protein, exhibited defective activation of NF-κB, or were sensitive to TNF-α-induced cell death. Islet cells, erythrocytes and liver cells of adult NOD mice did not exhibit the LMP2 defect. Thus, NOD mouse islets expresed LMP2 protein and do not exhibit increased sensitivity to TNF-α-induced apoptosis (Hayashi and Faustman, 1999). Dysfunction of a gene in the MHC region of the genome thus virtually abolishes the activity of a transcription factor that plays important roles in both immune and non-immune cellular functions. The NOD mouse thus represents a newly defined mosaic model of discordant MHC gene expression that exhibits marked proteasome dysfunction in an age- and tissue-specific manner.

The delayed maturation of lymphocytes and cytokine abnormalities apparent in NOD mouse that spontaneously develop type 1 diabetes are mirrored, in part, by the clinical phenotypes of knockout mice lacking NK-κB subunits or LMP2 (Beg and Baltimore, 1996; Beg et al., 1995; Caamano et al., 1998; Franzoso et al., 1997; Horwitz et al., 1997; Iotsova et al., 1997; Sha et al., 1995; Snapper et al., 1996; Van Kaer et al., 1994). The clinical relevance of the phenotypes of the NOD mouse and of these various knockout animals to human disease is supported by the existence of nearly identical cytokine and lymphocyte maturation defects in humans with type 1 diabetes (Crisa et al., 1992; Faustman et al., 1991a; Rabinovitch and Skyler, 1998).

In conclusion, these research findings have demonstrated the existence of a marked defect in proteasome function in lymphocytes from autoimmune diabetes-prone NOD mice. This dysfunction results from a lack of the LMP2 subunit, which is encoded by a gene located in the MHC region of the genome, and it results in both impaired processing of self-peptides for presentation by MHC class I molecules as well as the inability to activate NF-κB. A similar age-related defect in granulocytes-macrophages is proposed to confer target specificity in autoimmunity towards tissues with intact expression. Abnormal processing of intracellular proteins thus may contribute to the pathogenesis of type 1 diabetes.

Acknowledgment. We thank T. Maniatis for helpful comments on the manuscript. This work was supported by the Iacocca Foundation and grant RO1 DE11151 (to Dr Denise Faustman) from the National Institutes of Health.

REFERENCES

Akiyama K. Y., Yokota K. Y., Kagawa S., Shimbara N., Tamura T., Akioka H., Nothwang H. G., Noda C., Tanaka K. and Ichihara A. (1994): cDNA cloning and interferon γ down-regulation of proteasomal subunits X and Y. Science, **265**, 1231–1234.

Aldrich C. J., Ljunggren H. G., Van Kaer L., Ashton-Rickardt P. G., Tonegawa S. and Forman J. (1994): Positive selection of self- and alloreactive CD8+ T cells in TAP-1 mutant mice. Proc. Natl. Acad. Sci. USA, **91**, 6525–6528.

Atkinson M. A. and Leiter E. H. (1999): The NOD mouse model of type 1 diabetes: as good as it gets? Nat. Med., **5**, 601–604.

Baeuerle P. A. and Baltimore D. (1996): NF-kappa B: ten years after. Cell, **87**, 13–20.

Baldwin A. S. (1996): The NF-κB and IκB proteins: new discoveries and insights. Annu. Rev. Immunol., **12**, 141–179.

Beg A. A. and Baltimore D. (1996): An essential role for NF-kappaB in preventing TNF-alpha--induced cell death. Science, **274**, 782–784.

Beg A. A., Sha W. C., Bronson R. T., Ghosh S. and Baltimore D. (1995): Embryonic lethality and liver degeneration in mice lacking the relA component of NF-kappa B. Nature, **376**, 167–170.

Belich M. P., Glynne R. J., Senger G., Sheer D. and Trowsdale J. (1994): Proteasome components with reciprocal expression to that of the MHC-encoded LMP proteins. Curr. Biol., **4**, 769–776.

Belich M. P., Salmeron A., Johnston L. H. and Ley S. C. (1999): TPL-2 kinase regulates the proteolysis of the NF-kappaB-inhibitory protein NF-kappaB1 p105. Nature, **397**, 363–368.

Bohnline E., Lowenthal J. W., Siekevitz M., Franza B. R. and Greene W. C. (1988): The same inducible nuclear protein regulates mitogen activation of both the interleukin-2 receptor-alpha gene and type 1 HIV. Cell, **53**, 827–836.

Burkly L., Hession C., Ogata L., Reilly C., Marconi L. A., Olson D., Tizard R., Cate R. and Lo D. (1995): Expression of relB is required for the development of thymic medulla and dendritic cells. Nature, **373**, 531–536.

Bushdid P. B., Brantley D. M., Yull F. E., Blaeuer G. L., Hoffman L. H., Niswander L. and Kerr L. D. (1998): Inhibition of NF-κB activity results in disruption of the apical ectodermal ringe and aberrant limb morphogenesis. Nature, **392**, 615–618.

Caamano J. H., Rizzo C. A., Durham S. K., Barton D. S., Raventos-Suarez C., Snapper C. M. and Bravo R. (1998): Nuclear factor (NF)-kappa B2 (p100/p52) is required for normal splenic microarchitecture and B cell-mediated immune responses. J. Exp. Med., **187**, 185–196.

Coux O. and Goldberg A. L. (1998): Enzymes catalyzing ubiquitination and proteolytic processing of the p105 precursor of nuclear factor κB1. J. Biol. Chem., **273**, 8820–8828.

Coux O., Tanaka K. and Goldberg A. L. (1996): Structure and functions of the 20S and 26S proteasomes. Annu. Rev. Biochem., **65**, 801–847.

Crisa L., Mordes J. P. and Rossini A. A. (1992): Autoimmune diabetes mellitus in the BB rat. Diabetes Metab. Rev., **8**, 9–37.

Cross S. L., Halden N. F., Lenardo M. and Leonard W. J. (1989): Functionally distinct NF-kappa B binding sites in the immunoglobulin kappa and IL-2 receptor alpha chain genes. Science, **244**, 466–468.

Cui H., Matusi K., Omura S., Schaver S. L., Matulka R. A., Sonenshein G. E. and Ju S. T. (1997): Proteasome regulation of activation-induced T cell death. Proc. Natl. Acad. Sci. USA, **94**, 7515–7520.

Fan C. M. and Maniatis T. (1991): Generation of p50 subunit of NF-κB by processing of p105 through an ATP-dependent pathway. Nature, **354**, 395–398.

Faustman D., Eisenbarth G. and Daley J. (1989): Abnormal T lymphocyte subsets in type I diabetes mellitus: analysis with anti-2H4 and anti-4B4 antibodies. Diabetes, **38**, 1462–1468.

Faustman D., Li X., Lin H. Y., Fu Y., Eisenbarth G., Avruch J. and Guo J. (1991a): Linkage of faulty major histocompatibility complex class I to autoimmune diabetes. Science, **254**, 1756–1761.

Faustman D., Schoenfeld D. and Ziegler R. (1991b): T-lymphocyte changes linked to autoantibodies: Association of insulin autoantibodies with $CD4^+CD45R^+$ lymphocyte subpopulation in prediabetic subjects. Diabetes, **40**, 590–597.

Foulis A. K. (1987): C. L. Oakley lecture (1987). The pathogenesis of beta cell destruction in type I (insulin-dependent) diabetes mellitus. J. Pathol., **152**, 141–148.

Franzoso G., Carlson L., Xing L., Poljak L., Shores E. W., Brown K. D., Leonardi A., Tran T., Boyce B. F. and Siebenlist U. (1997): Requirement for NF-κB in osteolast and B-cell development. Genes Dev., **11**, 3482–3496.

Freland S., Chambers B. J., Andersson M., Van Kaer L. and Ljunggren H. G. (1998): Rejection of allogeneic and syngeneic but not MHC class I-deficient tumor grafts by MHC class I-deficient mice. J. Immunol., **160**, 572–579.

Fruh K., Yang Y., Arnold D., Chambers J., Wu L., Waters J. B., Spies T. and Peterson P. A. (1992): Alternative exon usage and processing of the major histocompatibility complex-encoded proteasome subunits. J. Biol. Chem., **267**, 22131–22140.

Fu Y., Nathan D. M., Li F., Li X. and Faustman D. L. (1993): Defective major histocompatibility complex class I expression on lymphoid cells in autoimmunity. J. Clin. Invest., **91**, 2301–2307.

Fu Y., Yan G., Shi L. and Faustman D. (1998): Antigen processing and autoimmunity. Evaluation of mRNA abundance and function of HLA-linked genes. Ann. NY Acad. Sci., **842**, 138–155.

Gaczynska M., Goldberg A. L., Tanaka K., Hendil K. B. and Rock K. L. (1996): Proteasome subunits X and Y alter peptidase activities in opposite ways to the interferon-gamma-induced subunits LMP2 and LMP7. J. Biol. Chem., **271**, 17275–17280.

Ghosh S. and Baltimore D. (1990): Activation *in vitro* of NF-κB by phosphorylation of its inhibitor IκB. Nature, **344**, 678–682.

Glas R., Ohlen C., Hoglund P. and Karre K. (1994): The $CD8^+$ T cell repertoire in β_2-microglobulin-deficient mice is biased towards reactivity against self-major histocompatibility complex class I. J. Exp. Med., **179**, 661–672.

Goldberg A. L. (1995): Functions of the proteasome: the lysis at the end of the tunnel. Science, **268**, 522–523.

Griffin T. A., Nandi D., Cruz M., Fehling H. J., Van Kaer L., Monaco J. J. and Colbert R. A. (1998): Immunoproteasome assembly: Cooperative incorporation of interferon γ (IFN-γ)-inducible subunits. J. Exp. Med., **187**, 97–104.

Hanafusa T., Miyazaki A., Miyagawa J., Tamura S., Inada M., Yamada K., Shinji Y., Katsura H., Yamagata K. and Itoh N. (1990): Examination of islets in the pancreas biopsy specimens from newly diagnosed type 1 (insulin-dependent) diabetic patients. Diabetologia, **33**, 105–111.

Hayashi T. and Faustman D. (1999): NOD mice are defective in proteasome production and activation of NF-κB. Mol. Cell. Biol., **19**, 8646–8659.

Hayashi T. and Faustman D. (2000): Essential role of HLA-encoded proteasome subunits in NF-κB activation and prevention of TNF-α induced apoptosis. J. Biol. Chem., **275**, 5238–5247.

Hayashi T., Sekine T. and Okamoto T. (1993a): Identification of a new serine kinase that activates NF-kappa B by direct phosphorylation. J. Biol. Chem., **268**, 26790–26795.

Hayashi T., Ueno Y. and Okamoto T. (1993b): Oxireductive regulation of nuclear factor κB, involvement of a cellular reducing catalyst thioredoxin. J. Biol. Chem., **268**, 11380–11388.

Hisamatsu H., Shimbara N., Saito Y., Kristensen P., Hendil K. B., Fujiwara T., Takahashi E., Tanahashi N., Tamura T., Ichihara A. and Tanaka K. (1996): Newly identified pair of proteasomal subunits regulated reciprocally by interferon-γ. J. Exp. Med., **183**, 1807–1816.

Horwitz B. H., Scott M. L., Cherry S. R., Bronson R. T. and Baltimore D. (1997): Failure of lymphopoiesis after adoptive transfer of NF-kappaB-deficient fetal liver cells. Immunity, **6**, 765–772.

Hu Y., Baud V., Delhase M., Zhang P., Deerinck T., Ellisman M., Johnson R. and Karin M. (1999): Abnormal morphogenesis but intact IKK activation in mice lacking the IKKα subunit of IκB kinase. Science, **284**, 316–320.

Iotsova V., Caamano J., Loy J., Yang Y., Lewin A. and Bravo R. (1997): Osteopetrosis in mice lacking NF-kappaB1 and NF-kappaB2. Nat. Med., **3**, 1285–1289.

Jansen A., Van Hagen M. and Drexhage H. A. (1995): Defective maturation and function of antigen-presenting cells in type I diabetes. Lancet, **345**, 491–492.

Kanegae Y., Ransone L. J., Wamsley P., Schmitt M. J., Boyer T. G., Zhou Q., Berk A. J. and Verma I. M. (1998): Role of Rel/NF-κB transcription factors during the outgrowth of the vertebrate limb. Nature, **392**, 611–614.

Kay T. W. H., Campbell I. L., Oxbrow L. and Harrison L. C. (1991): Overexpression of class I major histocompatibility complex accompanies insulitis in the nonobese diabetic mouse and is prevented by anti-interferon-γ antibody. Diabetologia, **34**, 779–785.

Kontgen F., Grumont R. J., Strasser A., Metcalf D., Li R., Tarlinton D. and Gerondakis S. (1995): Mice lacking the c-rel proto-oncogene exhibit defects in lymphocyte proliferation, humoral immunity, and interleukin-2 expression. Genes Dev., **9**, 1965–1977.

Li F., Hauser S. L., Linan M. J., Stein M. C. and Faustman D. L. (1995): Reduced expression of peptide-loaded HLA class I molecules on multiple sclerosis lymphocytes. Ann. Neurol., **38**, 147–154.

Li Q., Lu Q., Hwang J. Y., Buscher D., Lee K. F., Izpisua-Belmonte J. C. and Verma I. M. (1999a): IKK1-deficient mice exhibit abnormal development of skin and skeleton. Genes Dev., **13**, 1322–1328.

Li Q., Van Antwerp D., Mercurio F., Lee K. F. and Verma I. M. (1999b): Severe liver degeneration in mice lacking the IkappaB kinase 2 gene. Science, **284**, 321–325.

Li X. and Faustman D. (1993): Use of donor ß2-microglobulin-deficient transgenic mouse liver cells for isografts, allografts, and xenografts. Transplantation, **55**, 940–946.

Lin J., Tserng K., Chen C., Lin L. and Tung T. (1970): Abrin and ricin: new anti-tumor substances. Nature, **227**, 292–293.

Lin L., De Martino G. N. and Greene W. C. (1998): Co-translational biogenesis of NF-kappa B p50 by the 26S proteasome. Cell, **92**, 819–828.

MacKichan M. L., Logeat F. and Israel A. (1996): Phosphorylation of p105 PEST sequences via a Redox-insensitive pathway up-regulates processing of p50 NF-κB. J. Biol. Chem., **271**, 6084–6091.

Makino S., Kunimoto K., Muraoka Y., Mizushima Y., Katagiri K. and Tochino Y. (1980): Breeding of a non-obese, diabetic strain of mice. Jikken Dobutsu. Exp. Animals, **29**, 1–13.

Maniatis T. (1999): A ubiquitin ligase complex essential for the NF-kappaB, Wnt/Wingless, and Hedgehog signaling pathways. Genes Dev., **13**, 505–510.

Naumann N. and Scheidereit C. (1994): Activation of NF-κB *in vivo* is regulated by multiple phosphorylations. EMBO J., **13**, 4597–4607.

Neri A., Chang C. C., Lombardi L., Salina M., Corradini P., Maiolo A. T., Chaganti R. S. and Dalla-Favera R. (1991): B cell lymphoma-associated chromosomal translocation involves candidate oncogene lyt-10, homologous to NF-kappa B p50. Cell, **67**, 1075–1087.

Ono S. J., Issa-Chergui B., Colle E., Guttmann R. D., Seemayer T. A. and Fuks A. (1988): IDDM in BB rats. Enhanced MHC class I heavy-chain gene expression in pancreatic islets. Diabetes, **37**, 1411–1418.

Orian A., Whiteside S., Israel A., Stancovski I., Schwartz A. L. and Ciechanover A. (1995):

Ubiquitin-mediated processing of NF-kappa B transcriptional activator precursor p105. Reconstitution of a cell-free system and identification of the ubiquitin-carrier protein, E2, and a novel ubiquitin-protein ligase, E3, involved in conjugation. J. Biol. Chem., **270**, 21707–21714.

Pahl H. L. and Baeuerle P. A. (1996): Control of gene expression by proteolysis. Curr. Opin. Cell Biol., **8**, 340–347.

Palombella V., Rando O. J., Goldberg A. L. and Maniatis T. (1994): The ubiquitin-proteasome pathway is required for processing the NF-κB1 precursor protein and the activation of NF-κB. Cell, **78**, 773–785.

Rabinovitch A. and Skyler J. S. (1998): Prevention of type 1 diabetes. Med. Clin. North Am., **82**, 739–755.

Schmid R. M., Perkins N. D., Duckett C. S., Andrews P. C. and Nabel G. J. (1991): Cloning of an NF-kappa B subunit which stimulates HIV transcription in synergy with p65. Nature, **352**, 733–736.

Sears C., Olesen J., Rubin D., Finley D. and Maniatis T. (1998): NF-κB p105 processing via the ubiquitin-proteasome pathway. J. Biol. Chem., **273**, 1409–1419.

Sha W. C., Liou H. C., Tuomanen E. I. and Baltimore D. (1995): Targeted disruption of the p50 subunit of NF-kappa B leads to multifocal defects in immune responses. Cell, **80**, 321–330.

Smerdon R. A., Peakman M., Hussain M. J., Alviggi L., Watkins P. J., Leslie D. G. and Vergani D. (1993): Increase in simultaneous coexpression of naive and memory lymphocyte markers at diagnosis of IDDM. Diabetes, **42**, 127–133.

Snapper C. M., Zelazowski P., Rosas F. R., Kehry M. R., Tian M., Baltimore D. and Sha W. C. (1996): B cells from p50/NF-kappa B knockout mice have selective defects in proliferation, differentiation, germ-line CH transcription, and Ig class switching. J. Immunol., **156**, 183–191.

Stephens L. A., Thomas H. E. and Kay T. W. (1997): Protection of NIT-1 pancreatic beta-cells from immune attack by inhibition of NF-kappaB. J. Autoimmun., **10**, 293–298.

Sun S. C., Ganchi P. A., Beraud C., Ballard D. W. and Greene W. C. (1994): Autoregulation of the NF-kappa B transactivator RelA (p65) by multiple cytoplasmic inhibitors containing ankyrin motifs. Proc. Natl. Acad. Sci. USA, **91**, 1346–1350.

Takeda K., Takeuchi O., Tsujimura T., Itami S., Adachi O., Kawai T., Sanjo H., Yoshikawa K., Terada N. and Akira S. (1999): Limb and skin abnormalities in mice lacking IKKalpha. Science, **284**, 313–316.

Tan T. H., Huang G. P., Sica A., Ghosh P., Young H. A., Longo D. L. and Rice N. R. (1992): Kappa B site-dependent activation of the interleukin-2 receptor alpha-chain gene promoter by human C-Rel. Mol. Cell. Biol., **12**, 4067–4075.

Tanaka M., Fuentes M. E., Yamaguchi K., Durnin M. H., Dalrymple S. A., Hardy K. L. and Goeddel D. V. (1999): Embryonic lethality, liver degeneration, and impaired NF-kappa B activation in IKK-beta-deficient mice. Immunity, **10**, 421–429.

Thanos D. and Maniatis T. (1995): NF-kappa B: a lesson in family values. Cell, **80**, 529–532.

Van Antwerp D. J., Martin S. J., Kafri T., Green D. R. and Verma I. M. (1996): Suppression of TNF-alpha-induced apoptosis by NF-kappaB. Science, **274**, 787–789.

Van Kaer L., Ashton-Rickardt P. G., Eichelberger M., Gaczynska M., Nagashima K., Rock K. L., Goldberg A. L., Doherty P. C. and Tonegawa S. (1994): Altered peptidase and viral-specific T cell response in LMP-2 mutant mice. Immunity, **1**, 533–541.

Verma I. M., Stevenson E. M., Schwarz D. V., Antwerp S. and Miyamoto S. (1995): Rel/NF--kappa B/I kappa B family: intimate tales of association and dissociation. Genes Dev., **9**, 2723–2735.

Vidal-Puig A. and Faustman D. L. (1994): Tolerance to peripheral tissue is transient and maintained by tissue specific class I expression. Transplant. Proc., **26**, 3314–3316.

Vives-Pi M., Armengol M. P., Alcalde L., Costa M., Somoza N., Vargas F., Jaraquemada D. and Pujol-Borrell R. (1996): Expression of transporter associated with antigen processing-1 in the endocrine cells of human pancreatic islets: effect of cytokines and evidence of hyperexpression in IDDM. Diabetes, **45**, 779–788.

Wakatsuki Y., Neurath M. F., Max E. E. and Strober W. (1994): The B cell-specific transcription factor BSAP regulates B cell proliferation. J. Exp. Med., **179**, 1099–1108.

Wang C. Y., Mayo M. W. and Baldwin A. S. (1996): TNF and cancer therapy-induced apoptosis potentiation by inhibition of NF-kappaB. Science, **274**, 784–787.

Weih F., Carrasco D., Durham S. K., Barton D. S., Rizzo C. A., Ryseck R. P., Lira S. A. and Bravo R. (1995): Multiorgan inflammation and hematopoietic abnormalities in mice with a targeted disruption of RelB, a member of the NF-kappa B/Rel family. Cell, **80**, 331–340.

Weringer E. J. and Like A. A. (1988): Identification of T cell subsets and class I and class II antigen expression in islet grafts and pancreatic islets of diabetic BioBreeding/Worcester rats. Am. J. Pathol., **132**, 292–303.

Wu M., Lee H., Bellas R. E., Schauer S. L., Arsura M., Katz D., Fitzgerald M. J., Rothstein T. L., Sherr D. H. and Sonenshein G. E. (1996): Inhibition of NF-kappaB/Rel induces apoptosis of murine B cells. EMBO J., **15**, 4682–4690.

Yan G., Fu Y. and Faustman D. L. (1997): Reduced expression of *Tap1* and *Lmp2* antigen processing genes in the nonobese diabetic (NOD) mouse due to a mutation in their shared bidirectional promoter. J. Immunol., **159**, 3068–3080.

Yang X. D., Tisch R., Singer S. M., Cao Z. A., Liblau R. S., Schreiber R. D. and McDevitt H. O. (1994): Effect of tumor necrosis factor alpha on insulin-dependent diabetes mellitus in NOD mice. I. The early development of autoimmunity and the diabetogenic process. J. Exp. Med., **180**, 995–1004.

COMPLEMENT REGULATORY PROTEINS AND AUTOIMMUNITY

MITSUHIRO KAWANO

Second Department of Internal Medicine, School of Medicine, Kanazawa University, Kanazawa, Japan

Abstract To discriminate self from non-self is an essential issue in the immune system. Autologous cells are protected against complement-mediated cell injury by the self-recognition mechanism using complement regulatory proteins composed of complement receptor type 1 (CR1, CD35), membrane cofactor protein (MCP, CD46), decay accelerating factor (DAF, CD55) and homologous restriction factor (protectin, CD59). Recently, the up-regulation of these molecules has been widely shown in inflammatory tissues and organs affected by autoimmune diseases, and *in vitro* assays have revealed that immune complexes or several cytokines, including interferon γ, tumor necrosis factor α, interleukin 1β and transforming growth factor β, can up-regulate these molecules. In contrast, it has been found that expression of these complement regulatory proteins is markedly decreased on autologous cells undergoing apoptosis. These findings suggest that complement regulatory proteins have dual roles at inflammatory sites: enhancement of cellular resistance to complement attack and acceleration of the clearance of cells injurious to the organism due to complement-mediated mechanisms. To assist the former function, a therapeutic approach using recombinant soluble complement regulatory proteins may provide a promising strategy for the treatment of autoimmune diseases.

Key words: membrane cofactor protein (CD46); decay accelerating factor (CD55); homologous restriction factor (CD59); complement receptor type 1 (CD35).

1. INTRODUCTION

New approaches to the treatment of autoimmune diseases are being actively sought. In this review, I outline one such promising approach that has been suggested by recent advances in the study of basic immunology. In the course of the evolution of the immune system, discrimination of self from infectious and other non-self was very important (Atkinson and Farries, 1987; Janeway, 1992). The alternative complement pathway is a primitive

A. Górski et al. (eds.), Autoimmunity, 73–82.

and non-adoptive immune response system which distinguishes self from non-self immediately and attacks non-self through the formation of the membrane attack complex (MAC) (Atkinson and Farries, 1987; Janeway, 1992). At the first step of the alternative pathway, C3 is deposited on the surface of non-self followed by activation of a subsequent complement cascade and MAC perforates the target cells (Roitt, 1997). In addition, released C3a and C5a, which are products cleaved by C3 and C5 convertases (C3bBb), dilate capillaries and increase vascular permeability to assemble neutrophils in the inflammatory site (Roitt, 1997). On the other hand, normal human cells are resistant to complement-mediated lysis by mechanisms using a special self-recognition system. This system is composed of specific membrane-bound proteins such as decay accelerating factor (DAF, CD55) (Nicholson-Weller et al., 1982), membrane cofactor protein (MCP, CD46) (Cole et al., 1985; Seya et al., 1986) and homologous restriction factor (protectin, CD59) (Davies et al., 1989). Complement receptor type 1 (CR1, CD35) (Hebert, 1987) is also involved in the regulation of C3 fragment deposition. Neoplastic cells are also protected from autologous complement-mediated cell injury by these complement regulatory proteins (Brasoveanu et al., 1997; Cheung et al., 1988; Seya et al., 1990). In contrast, the absence of these molecules on tumor cells makes them susceptible to complement attack (Brasoveanu et al., 1997; Cheung et al., 1988; Seya et al., 1990).

2. COMPLEMENT REGULATORY PROTEINS

The inhibitory points of the complement activation cascade are different in each protein (Table 1). CD46 and CD55 block C3b deposition on the autologous cell surface (Cole et al., 1985; Nicholson-Weller et al., 1982; Seya et al., 1986). CD46 acts as a cofactor for the factor I-mediated cleavage of the

Table 1. Function of complement regulatory proteins

CD no.	Other name(s)	Function
CD35	Complement receptor 1 (CR1)	Complement inhibitor of classical and alternative pathway
CD46	Membrane cofactor protein (MCP)	Cofactor for factor I-mediated cleavage of the C3b and C4b
CD55	Decay-accelerating factor (DAF)	Acceleration of the dissociation of C3 and C5 convertases
CD59	Homologous restriction factor (HRF-20), protectin	Inhibition of membrane attack complex

activated complement components C3b and C4b (Cole et al., 1985; Seya et al., 1986). CD55 accelerates the dissociation of C3bBb and limits amplification of the complement cascade (Nicholson-Weller et al., 1982). CD59 influences the later step of the alternative pathway, where CD59 interferes with C9 incorporation into C3b-8 complex (Davies et al., 1989). CD55 and CD59 are glycosylphosphatidylinositol (GPI)-anchored proteins, the absence of which is pathogenetically essential and clinically important in paroxysmal nocturnal hemoglobinuria (PNH) (Jarva and Meri, 1999).

3. SOLUBLE FORMS OF COMPLEMENT REGULATORY PROTEINS

Although complement regulatory proteins are membrane-bound proteins and usually act on autologous cell surfaces, soluble forms of each molecule are detected in serum, saliva, tear, urine and other body fluids (Hara et al., 1992; Lehto et al., 1995; Medof et al., 1987; Rooney and Morgan, 1992; Seya et al., 1995). The serum levels of these soluble molecules, however, are not sufficient to control complement attack on the affected organs (Kawano et al., 1999). So the measurement of soluble complement regulatory proteins is useful merely to estimate local inflammation with complement involvement. Moreover, some neoplasms are also known to influence serum levels of these soluble complement regulatory proteins by shedding these molecules from their surfaces (Brasoveanu et al., 1997).

4. AUTOIMMUNITY AND COMPLEMENT SYSTEM

In autoimmune disease, the targeted tissue is destroyed mainly by autoreactive T cells or immune complex-mediated tissue damage. It is widely accepted that the complement system is also involved in the uncontrolled self-toxic immune system in autoimmune diseases (Falk et al., 1985; Garwryl et al., 1988; Schur, 1997). Immune complexes formed in the blood or directly on the affected tissues induce activation of the complement system (Gauthier and Emlen, 1997). As a reflection of *in vivo* complement activation, decreased serum complement levels form a distinct feature of active systemic lupus erythematosus (SLE). Hence, a better understanding of complement regulatory proteins in active and inactive SLE or other autoimmune diseases may provide new insights into the role of complement system abnormalities in autoimmunity.

5. REGULATION OF COMPLEMENT REGULATORY PROTEINS IN INFLAMMATORY TISSUES

The amounts of these complement regulatory proteins on cell surfaces are influenced by a variety of inflammatory situations and regulated by many chemical mediators. *In vitro* assays using cultured tumor cell lines or normal cultured human keratinocytes revealed that interferon γ (IFN-γ), tumor necrosis factor α (TNF-α), interleukin 1β (IL-1β) and transforming growth factor β (TGF-β) can up-regulate these molecules, with the type of protein up-regulated differing according to the individual cell type (Bjorge et al., 1995; Pasch et al., 1999; Schmitt et al., 1999). Mason et al. (1999) showed that the amount of CD55 expression on cultured human endothelial cells was increased by TNF-α and IFN-γ, but this was not true of CD46 or CD59. Shibata et al. (1991) demonstrated that immune complex formation and complement activation *in vitro* significantly increased CD55 expression on the mesangial cells. Phorbol-12-myristate-13 acetate (PMA) and calcium ionophore were also shown to induce up-regulation of CD59 on a cultured human endothelial cell line (Meri et al., 1993). In lupus nephritis, increased expression of CD59 (Tamai et al., 1991) and CD46 (Endoh et al., 1993) has been reported on glomerular endothelial cells and mesangial cells, where C3b/C3c deposition occurs. Circulating sCD46 was also increased in active SLE and decreased with control of the disease activity (Kawano et al., 1999). Similarly, up-regulated expression of CD46, CD55 and CD59 was detected on the acinar and ductal epithelial cells in Sjögren's syndrome (SS) and high concentrations of soluble CD55 and CD59 have been shown in saliva from SS patients (Cuida et al., 1997). In inflammatory joints of rheumatoid arthritis (RA) patients, these three molecules are strongly stained on the chondrocyte surfaces and their up-regulation is observed if cultured chondrocytes are stimulated with IL-1 (Davies et al., 1994). It was also shown that the neutrophils in the synovial fluid (SF) from patients with RA possessed an increased amount of CD55 as compared to those in peripheral blood (Jones et al., 1994). In these diseases, although complement regulatory proteins are originally localized at normal tissues (Bardenstein et al., 1994; Guc et al., 1993; Nose et al., 1990; Rooney et al., 1991), the up-regulation of these molecules at affected organs may imply a common protective response against unexpected attack by the complement system. These observations suggest that, in the self-destructive processes of autoimmune disease, each cell of the affected organ resists complement attack through up-regulation of cell surface-bound complement regulatory proteins.

6. REGULATION OF COMPLEMENT REGULATORY PROTEINS ON APOPTOTIC CELL SURFACES

On the other hand, the involvement of the complement system in apoptotic cells has also been noted recently (Matsui et al., 1994; Tsuji et al., 1994). In the course of apoptotic cell death of activated lymphocytes, these cells need first to be recognized as non-self with the apoptotic cells then cleared by phagocytes. The molecular mechanisms by which cells undergoing apoptosis are recognized and eliminated by phagocytes include thrombospondin (TSP) – TSP receptor (α v β3 integrin and CD36) interaction, phosphatidylserine (PS) – PS receptor interaction, CD14-mediated recognition and lectin-mediated recognition (Devitt et al., 1998; Savill et al., 1993). In addition, reduced expression of these complement regulatory proteins has been reported on the surface of apoptotic cells (Matsui et al., 1994). Tsuji et al. (1994) reported that the amount of CD46, CD55 and CD59 on apoptotic human umbilical vein endothelial cells (HUVEC) decreased in each case to about half of that on intact HUVEC. Reduced expression of CD46 and CD55 inducing attachment of C3b on the surface of apoptotic cells resulted in formation of iC3b, a ligand of the complement receptor type 3 (CR3) of phagocytes (Matsui et al., 1994; Tsuji et al., 1994). In contrast, diminished CD59 implies susceptibility to complement-mediated cell lysis rather than apoptosis. However, sublytic MAC attack is thought to activate target cells in producing potential inflammatory mediators including oxidant products (Morgan, 1989). Although the detailed mechanism is unclear, target cell injury induced by sublytic MAC attack may be also involved in the process of apoptotic autologous cell clearance.

Epstein-Barr virus (EBV)-associated infectious mononucleosis (IM) is a well-analyzed acute viral infection, in which activation-induced cell death plays an important role in the clearance of activated $CD8^+$ T lymphocytes (Uehara et al., 1992). In this disease, decreased expression of CD59 was detected in an activated $CD8^+$ subpopulation of peripheral T lymphocytes, and these $CD59^{dim}CD8^+$ T cells were more susceptible to apoptosis than $CD59^{bright}CD8^+$ T cells (Kawano et al., 1997). Although whether decreased CD59 is involved in apoptotic lymphocyte clearance is unclear, this finding suggests that decreased expression of CD59 on $CD8^+$ T cells may discriminate the susceptibility of activated $CD8^+$ T cells to activation-induced cell death. A similar $CD59^{dim}CD8^+$ T cell subpopulation, more likely to undergo apoptosis when cultured *in vitro* without any growth factors, has been detected in a group of active SLE patients (Tsunoda et al., 2000). Jones and Morgan (1995) analyzed apoptotic polymorphonuclear leukocytes (PMN) and found a marked reduction in cell surface expression of CD59 and CD55, but not of

CD46 on PMN. These findings suggest that decreased expression of complement regulatory proteins is a common feature of cells undergoing apoptosis and has an important role in the clearance of cells undergoing apoptosis.

7. CLINICAL APPLICATION OF COMPLEMENT REGULATORY PROTEINS

To control complement-mediated autologous cell injury, soluble forms of complement regulatory proteins may provide useful therapeutic tools. An analysis of the function of recombinant soluble CD55 (rsCD55) revealed complement activation inhibiting activity in the fluid phase of this protein (Moran et al., 1992). Christiansen et al. (1996) showed that rsCD35 was the most effective soluble complement regulatory protein at regulating both classical and alternative pathway activation and rsCD46 was as effective as rsCD35 in inhibiting the alternative pathway. Recombinant soluble CD59 is also useful in regulating complement attack (Sugita et al., 1994) and has been applied to protect against hyperacute rejection in xenotransplantation (Kennedy et al., 1994). Soluble CD59, however, is not as effective as other soluble complement regulatory proteins (rsCD35, rsCD46 and rsCD55), especially in the presence of serum, because it needs to be positioned close to the site of MAC formation (Kennedy et al., 1994; Sugita et al., 1994; Zhang et al., 1999). Hence, a specific antigen targeting antibody-CD59 fusion protein has been produced to supply soluble CD59 function at inflammatory sites (Zhang et al., 1999). Transfection of CD59 on cells also protects them from MAC attack and over-expression of complement regulatory proteins has shown therapeutic feasibility (Nangaku et al., 1996).

In summary, control of the activation of the complement system using recombinant soluble complement regulatory proteins is one promising strategy for the treatment of autoimmune diseases. If exaggerated complement reactions characteristic of these diseases can be selectively regulated using complement regulatory proteins without influencing the normal complement activation in inflammatory sites, then clinical application of these molecules in autoimmune diseases should become a clinical reality in the future. It is hoped that the information provided in this review will encourage further investigation of this field.

Acknowledgment. I thank Drs. H. Mabuchi, I. Koni, H. Muramoto and T. Seya for helpful advice, and Mr. J. S. Gelblum for a critical reading of the manuscript.

REFERENCES

Atkinson J. P. and Farries T. (1987): Separation of self from non-self in the complement system. Immunol. Today, **8**, 212–215.

Bardenstein D. S., Dietz Y., Lass J. H. and Medof M. E. (1994): Localization of the complement membrane attack complex inhibitor (CD59) in human conjunctiva and lacrimal gland. Curr. Eye Res., **13**, 851–855.

Bjorge L., Jensen T. S., Ulvestad E., Vedeler C. A. and Matre R. (1995): The influence of tumor necrosis factor-α, interleukin-1β and interferon-γ on the expression and function of the complement regulatory protein CD59 on the human colonic adenocarcinoma cell line HT29. Scand. J. Immunol., **41**, 350–356.

Brasoveanu L. I., Fonsatti E., Visintin A., Pavlovic M., Cattarossi I., Colizzi F., Gasparollo A., Coral S., Horejsi V., Altomonte M. and Maio M. (1997): Melanoma cells constitutively release an anchor-positive soluble form of protectin (sCD59) that retains functional activities in homologous complement-mediated cytotoxicity. J. Clin. Invest., **100**, 1248–1255.

Cheung N. V., Walter E. I., Smith-Mensah W. H., Ratnoff W. D., Tykocinski M. L. and Medof M. E. (1988): Decay-accelerating factor protects human tumor cells from complement-mediated cytotoxicity *in vitro*. J. Clin. Invest., **81**, 1122–1128.

Christiansen D., Milland J., Thorley B. R., McKenzie I. F. C. and Loveland B. E. (1996): A functional analysis of recombinant soluble CD46 *in vivo* and a comparison with recombinant soluble forms of CD55 and CD35 *in vitro*. Eur. J. Immunol., **26**, 578–585.

Cole J. L., Housley G. A. jr., Dykman T. R., MacDermott R. P. and Atkinson J. P. (1985): Identification of an additional class of C3-binding membrane proteins of human peripheral blood leukocytes and cell lines. Proc. Natl. Acad. Sci. USA, **82**, 859–863.

Cuida M., Legler D. W., Eidsheim M. and Jonsson R. (1997): Complement regulatory proteins in the salivary glands and saliva of Sjögren's syndrome patients and healthy subjects. Clin. Exp. Rheumatol., **15**, 615–623.

Davies A., Simmons D. L., Hale G., Harrison R. A., Tighe H., Lachmann P. J. and Waldmann H. (1989): CD59, an LY-6-like protein expressed in human lymphoid cells, regulates the action of the complement membrane attack complex on homologous cells. J. Exp. Med., **170**, 637–654.

Davies M. E., Horner A., Loveland B. E. and McKenzie I. F. C. (1994): Upregulation of complement regulators MCP (CD46), DAF (CD55) and protectin (CD59) in arthritic joint disease. Scand. J. Rheumatol., **23**, 316–321.

Devitt A., Moffatt O. D., Raykundalia C., Capra J. D., Simmons D. L. and Gregory C. D. (1998): Human CD14 mediates recognition and phagocytosis of apoptotic cells. Nature, **392**, 505–509.

Endoh M., Yamashina M., Ohi H., Funahashi K., Ikuno T., Yasugi T., Atkinson J. P. and Okada H. (1993): Immunohistochemical demonstration of membrane cofactor protein (MCP) of complement in normal and diseased kidney tissues. Clin. Exp. Immunol., **94**, 182–188.

Falk R. J., Dalmasso A. P., Kim Y., Lam S. and Michael A. (1985): Radioimmunoassay of the attack complex of complement in serum from patients with systemic lupus erythematosus. N. Engl. J. Med., **315**, 1584–1589.

Garwryl M. A., Chudwin D. S., Longlois P. F. and Lint T. F. (1988): The terminal complement complex, C5b-9, a marker of disease activity in patients with systemic lupus erythematosus. Arthritis Rheum., **31**, 188–195.

Gauthier V. J. and Emlen J. W. (1997): Immune complexes in systemic lupus erythematosus. In Wallace D. J. and Hahn B. H.: Dubois' lupus erythematosus. 5th ed. Williams & Wilkins, Baltimore–Philadelphia–London–Paris–Bangkok–Buenos Aires–Hong Kong–Munich–Sydney –Tokyo–Wrocław, 207–220.

Guc D., Gulati P., Lemercier C., Lappin D., Birnie G. D. and Whaley K. (1993): Expression of the components and regulatory proteins of the alternative complement pathway and the membrane attack complex in normal and diseased synovium. Rheumatol. Int., **13**, 139–146.

Hara T., Kuriyama S., Kiyohara H., Nagase Y., Matsumoto M. and Seya T. (1992): Soluble forms of membrane cofactor protein (CD46, MCP) are present in plasma, tears, and seminal fluid in normal subjects. Clin. Exp. Immunol., **89**, 490–494.

Hebert L. A. (1987): Clearance of immune complexes from the circulation of man and other primates. Am. J. Kidney Dis., **17**, 352–361.

Janeway C. A. Jr. (1992): The immune system evolved to discriminate infectious nonself from noninfectious self. Immunol. Today, **13**, 11–16.

Jarva H. and Meri S. (1999): Paroxysmal nocturnal haemoglobinuria: the disease and a hypothesis for a new treatment. Scand. J. Immunol., **49**, 119–125.

Jones J., Laffafian I., Cooper A. M., Williams B. D. and Morgan B. P. (1994): Expression of complement regulatory molecules and other surface markers on neutrophils from synovial fluid and blood of patients with rheumatoid arthritis. Br. J. Rheumatol., **33**, 707–712.

Jones J. and Morgan B. P. (1995): Apoptosis is associated with reduced expression of complement regulatory molecules, adhesion molecules and other receptors on polymorphonuclear leucocytes: functional relevance and role in inflammation. Immunology, **86**, 651–660.

Kawano M., Seya T., Koni I. and Mabuchi H. (1999): Elevated serum levels of soluble membrane cofactor protein (CD46, MCP) in patients with systemic lupus erythematosus (SLE). Clin. Exp. Immunol., **116**, 542–546.

Kawano M. Tsunoda S., Koni I., Mabuchi H., Muramoto H., Yachie A. and Seki H. (1997): Decreased expression of 20-kD homologous restriction factor (HRF20, CD59) on T lymphocytes in Epstein-Barr virus (EBV)-induced infectious mononucleosis. Clin. Exp. Immunol., **108**, 260–265.

Kennedy S. P., Rollins S. A., Burton W. V., Sims P. J., Bothwell A. L. M., Squinto S. P. and Zavoico G. B. (1994): Protection of porcine aortic endothelial cells from complement-mediated cell lysis and activation by recombinant human CD59. Transplantation, **57**, 1494–1501.

Lehto T., Honkanen E., Teppo A. M. and Meri S. (1995): Urinary excretion of protectin (CD59), complement SC5b-9 and cytokines in membranous glomerulonephritis. Kidney Int., **47**, 1403–1411.

Mason J. C., Yarwood H., Sugars K., Morgan B. P., Davies K. A. and Haskard D. O. (1999): Induction of decay-accelerating factor by cytokines or the membrane-attack complex protects vascular endothelial cells against complement deposition. Blood, **94**, 1673–1682.

Matsui H., Tsuji S., Nishimura H. and Nagasawa S. (1994): Activation of the alternative pathway of complement by apoptotic Jurkat cells. FEBS Lett., **351**, 419–422.

Medof M. E., Walter E. I., Rutgers J. L., Knowles D. M. and Nussenzweig V. (1987): Identification of the complement decay-accelerating factor (DAF) on epithelium and glandular cells and in body fluids. J. Exp. Med., **165**, 848–864.

Meri S., Mattila P. and Renkonen R. (1993): Regulation of CD59 expression on human endothelial cell line E. A. hy 926. Eur. J. Immunol., **23**, 2511–2516.

Moran P., Beasley H., Gorrell A., Martin E., Gribling P., Fuchs H., Gillett N., Burton L. E. and Caras I. W. (1992): Human recombinant soluble decay accelerating factor inhibits complement activation *in vitro* and *in vivo*. J. Immunol., **149**, 1736–1743.

Morgan B. P. (1989): Complement membrane attack on nucleated cells: resistance, recovery and non-lethal effect. Biochem. J., **264**, 1–14.

Nangaku M., Meek R. L., Pippin J., Gordon K. L., Morgan B. P., Johnson R. J. and Couser W. G. (1996): Transfected CD59 protects mesangial cells from injury induced by antibody and complement. Kidney Int., **50**, 257–266.

Nicholson-Weller A., Burge J., Fearon D. T., Weller P. F. and Austen K. F. (1982): Isolation of a human erythrocyte membrane glycoprotein with decay-accelerating activity for C3 convertase of the complement system. J. Immunol., **129**, 184–189.

Nose M., Katoh M., Okada N., Kyogoku M. and Okada H. (1990): Tissue distribution of HRF 20, a novel factor preventing the membrane attack of homologous complement, and its predominant expression on endothelial cells *in vivo*. Immunology, **70**, 145–149.

Pasch M. C., Bos J. D., Daha M. R. and Asghar S. S. (1999): Transforming growth factor-beta isoforms regulate the surface expression of membrane cofactor protein (CD46) and CD59 on human keratinocytes. Eur. J. Immunol., **29**, 100–108.

Roitt I. M. (1997): Roitt's essential immunology. 9th ed. Blackwell Science, London, 3–21.

Rooney I. A., Davies A., Griffiths D., Williams J. D., Davies M., Meri S., Lachmann P. J. and Morgan B. P. (1991): The complement-inhibiting protein, protectin (CD59 antigen), is present and functionally active on glomerular epitherial cells. Clin. Exp. Immunol., **83**, 251–256.

Ronney I. A. and Morgan B. P. (1992): Characterization of the membrane attack complex inhibitory protein CD59 antigen on human amniotic cells and in amniotic fluid. Immunology, **76**, 541–547.

Savill J., Fadok V., Henson P. and Haslett C. (1993): Phagocyte recognition of cells undergoing apoptosis. Immunol. Today, **14**, 131–136.

Schmitt C. A., Schwaeble W., Wittig B. M., Meyer zum Buschenfelde K. H. and Dippold W. G. (1999): Expression and regulation by interferon-gamma on the membrane-bound complement regulators CD46 (MCP), CD55 (DAF) and CD59 in gastrointestinal tumours. Eur. J. Cancer, **35**, 117–124.

Schur P. H. (1997): Complement and systemic lupus erythematosus. In Wallace D. J. and Hahn B. H.: Dubois' lupus erythematosus. 5th ed. Williams & Wilkins, Baltimore–Philadelphia–London–Paris–Bangkok–Buenos Aires–Hong Kong–Munich–Sydney–Tokyo–Wrocław, 245–261.

Seya T., Hara T., Iwata K., Kuriyama S., Hasegawa T., Nagase Y., Miyagawa S., Matsumoto M., Hatanaka M. and Atkinson J. P. (1995): Purification and functional properties of soluble forms of membrane cofactor protein (MCP, CD46) of complement: Identification of forms increased in cancer patients' sera. Int. Immunol., **7**, 727–736.

Seya T., Hara T., Matsumoto M., Sugita Y. and Akedo H. (1990): Complement-mediated tumor cell damage induced by antibodies against membrane cofactor protein (MCP, CD46). J. Exp. Med., **172**, 1673–1680.

Seya T., Turner J. R. and Atkinson J. P. (1986): Purification and characterization of a membrane protein (gp45-70) which is a cofactor for cleavage of C3b and C4b. J. Exp. Med., **163**, 837–855.

Shibata T., Cosio F. G. and Birmingham D. J. (1991): Complement activation induces the expression of decay-acceleration factor on human mesangial cells. J. Immunol., **147**, 3901–3908.

Sugita Y., Ito K., Shiozuka K., Suzuki H., Gushima H., Tomita M. and Masuho Y. (1994): Recombinant soluble CD59 inhibits reactive hemolysis with complement. Immunology, **82**, 34–41.

Tamai H., Matsuo S., Fukatsu A., Nishikawa K., Sakamoto N., Yoshioka K., Okada N. and Okada H. (1991): Localization of 20-kD homologous restriction factor (HRF20) in diseased human glomeruli. An immunofluorescence study. Clin. Exp. Immunol., **84**, 256–262.

Tsuji S., Kaji K. and Nagasawa S. (1994): Activation of the alternative pathway of human complement by apoptotic human umbilical vein endothelial cells. J. Biochem., **116**, 794–800.

Tsunoda S., Kawano M., Koni I., Kasahara Y., Yachie A., Miyawaki T. and Seki H. (2000): Diminished expression of CD59 on activated $CD8^+$ T cells Undergoing apoptosis in SLE and Sjögren's syndrome. Scand. J. Immunol., **51**, 293–299.

Uehara T., Miyawaki T., Ohta K., Tamaru Y., Yokoi T., Nakamura S. and Taniguchi N. (1992): Apoptotic cell death of primed CD45RO+ T lymphocytes in Epstein-Barr virus-induced infectious mononucleosis. Blood, **80**, 452–458.

Zhang H., Yu J., Bajwa E., Morrison S. L. and Tomlinson S. (1999): Targeting of functional antibody-CD59 fusion proteins to a cell surface. J. Clin. Invest., **103**, 55–61.

PATHOGENIC IMMUNITY IN THEILER'S VIRUS-INDUCED DEMYELINATING DISEASE: A VIRAL MODEL FOR MULTIPLE SCLEROSIS

BYUNG S. KIM[1], JOANN P. PALMA[1], ATSUSHI INOUE[2] and CHANG-SUNG KOH[2]

[1] *Departments of Microbiology-Immunology and Pathology, Northwestern University Medical School, Chicago, IL 60611, USA*
[2] *Third Department of Internal Medicine, Shinshu University School of Medicine, Matsumoto 390, Japan*

Abstract Multiple sclerosis involves inflammatory immune responses in the central nervous system (CNS) and is considered as an autoimmune disease potentially associated with viral infection. The majority of experimental models rely heavily on the autoimmune components since similar diseases can be induced following immunization with various myelin antigens. A very attractive alternative model is the Theiler's murine encephalomyelitis virus-induced demyelinating disease. This disease is primarily a CD4+ T cell-mediated, inflammatory demyelinating disease induced following viral infection. Virus-specific inflammatory Th1 cell responses, rather than cytotoxic T lymphocyte response, play a critical role in the pathogenic immune responses. The major pathogenic epitopes have been identified and these are correlated with a Th1 type response to the epitopes following viral infection. In addition, the initial virus-specific immune response is followed by the autoimmune responses to myelin antigens. Assessment of cytokines produced locally in the CNS during the course of disease suggests involvement of inflammatory cytokines in the disease. Furthermore, the manipulation of inflammatory cytokine levels by administration of either recombinant cytokines or antibodies to the cytokines strongly influences the induction and/or progression of disease, supporting the importance of these inflammatory cytokines in this virus-induced demyelinating disease.

Key words: multiple sclerosis; Theiler's virus; demyelinating disease.

Abbreviations used: MS – multiple sclerosis, TMEV – Theiler's murine encephalomyelitis virus, CNS – central nervous system, Th – helper T lymphocytes, CTL – cytotoxic T lymphocytes, MHC – major histocompatibility complex, IDD – immune-mediated demyelinating disease, LPS – lipopolysaccharide.

A. Górski et al. (eds.), Autoimmunity, 83–94.

1. INTRODUCTION

Multiple sclerosis (MS) is a neurological disease characterized by demyelination in the white matter of the brain and spinal cord mediated by inflammatory immune responses (Adams and Victor, 1977). The clinical symptoms range from a mild nervous system disability to a severe degenerative paralyzing disorder. Because of the relatively high incidence and chronic nature of the disease, social and economic loss due to it is enormous. Although the cause of MS is unknown, one or more infectious agents may be involved in the initial tissue damage leading to autoimmunity (Johnson, 1975; McFarlin and McFarland, 1982; Soldan et al., 1997). Several virus-induced and autoimmune models have been used to study the pathogenic mechanisms of this disease (Alford et al., 1984; Dal Canto et al., 1996; Daniels et al., 1952; Miller et al., 1997). Among these experimental model systems, Theiler's murine encephalomyelitis virus (TMEV)-induced demyelination provides an excellent infectious model for MS (Dal Canto et al., 1996; Miller et al., 1997).

TMEV is a common enteric pathogen in mice and belongs to the *Picornaviridae* (Lipton and Friedmann, 1980; Theiler and Gard, 1940). The TMEV genome is encapsulated in an icosahedral capsid structure composed of 60 units of four capsid proteins (VP1, VP2, VP3 and VP4) (Lipton and Friedmann, 1980; Theiler and Gard, 1940). There are two major subgroups of TMEV: the GDVII and FA, viruses causing rapid fatal encephalitis, and the BeAn and DA strains, which result in a biphasic neurological disease in susceptible mice (Dal Canto et al., 1996). An intracerebral inoculation of TMEV DA or BeAn into susceptible mice results in a chronic immune-mediated demyelinating disease (IDD) that shares many of the features of human MS. Although undetectable with BeAn, the early acute phase of infection with DA displays flaccid limb paralysis and degeneration of neurons. On the other hand, a chronic inflammatory demyelination is characteristic of the late phase disease in both DA and BeAn infections. In addition, demyelination is primarily associated with cell-mediated immune responses and strong autoimmunity to myelin antigens is induced following the initial demyelination by virus-specific T cells (Miller et al., 1997).

2. PATHOGENIC EFFECT OF CD4$^+$ T CELL RESPONSES

Treatment with antibodies to either the class II or CD4 molecules suppressed demyelination induced by TMEV (Rodriguez et al., 1986; Welsh et al., 1987), strongly suggesting that the Th cell response is involved in the pathogenesis of demyelination. Subcutaneous immunization with UV-inactivated TMEV prior to, but not after, viral infection efficiently protects susceptible mice from demyelinating disease (Yahikozawa et al., 1997). The immune components involved in the protection/pathogenesis have been further analyzed by utilizing various fusion proteins containing individual viral capsid proteins or synthetic peptides representing antibody and/or T cell epitope regions. The locations of the major Th epitopes and linear antibody epitopes are diagrammatically shown in Fig. 1.

The majority of MHC class II-restricted helper T cell lines/clones derived from demyelinating lesions of the spinal cords after viral infection react with VP1 or VP2 fusion protein, suggesting that these virus-specific Th cells in the CNS are involved in the pathogenicity (Yauch and Kim, 1994). In addition, the majority of T cells (~90%) appear to recognize one of three predominant epitopes ($VP1_{233\text{-}250}$, $VP2_{74\text{-}86}$ and $VP3_{24\text{-}37}$), one on each major external capsid protein (Yauch et al., 1995). It is interesting to note that the VP3 Th epitope overlaps with the major VP3 linear antibody epitope (Fig. 1). Although the T cell responses to the three predominant epitopes are similar throughout the disease course, the level of IFN-γ production was highest in response to VP1, intermediate with VP2 and lowest with the VP3 epitope peptide (Yauch et al., 1998). Conversely, the production of Th2 cytokines is highest in response to VP3 and lowest following stimulation with VP1 epitope peptides. Preferential induction of the Th2 response by the VP3 epitope may be influenced by the overlap with a major antibody epitope (Yauch et al., 1998). Further immunization with the epitope peptides indicated that the $VP1_{233\text{-}250}$ and $VP2_{74\text{-}86}$ epitopes exacerbate the disease while the $VP3_{24\text{-}37}$ epitope does not. Moreover, most of the T cell clones derived from affected spinal cords produced IL-2 and IFN-γ, but not IL-4, suggesting that the majority of Th

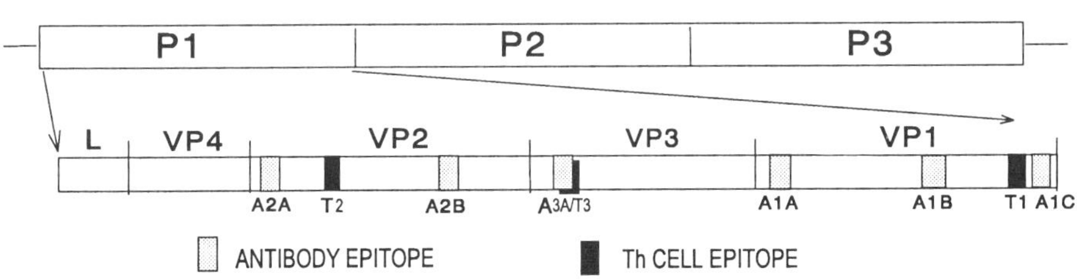

Figure 1. Viral genomic structure and the major epitopes for antibody as well as Th cells are schematically shown. VP1, VP2 and VP3 of Theiler's virus are external capsid proteins. Six major linear antibody epitopes and three Th epitopes have been found. These three Th epitopes, one on each external capsid protein, represent the great majority (~90%) of Th responses to TMEV

cells in the CNS is Th1 (Palma et al., 1996; Yauch and Kim, 1994; Yauch et al., 1998). In addition, the production of Th1 cytokine messages in the CNS preceded that of Th2 cytokine messages in virus-infected SJL mice, suggesting that the initial establishment of a Th1 response is critical for the pathogenesis of TMEV-induced demyelination. Taken together, these experiments strongly suggest that $CD4^+$ helper T cells are primarily involved in the pathogenesis of TMEV-IDD, in particular inflammatory Th1 responses to the VP1 and VP2 epitopes.

A spontaneous non-pathogenic variant virus displayed a single substitution of lysine to arginine at position 244 within the $VP1_{233\text{-}250}$ epitope (Fig. 1), which is the only amino acid difference found in the P1 region encoding all of the capsid proteins (Kim et al., 1998). The overall T cell response to the variant virus is primarily Th2 type, whereas that induced after infection with the wild type is Th1 type (unpublished data). Thus, such a spontaneous single amino acid change in a predominant Th epitope of a viral coat protein may be able to exert a profound impact on the type of Th response determining the pathogenicity of a virus, hence altering the outcome of disease.

The T cell repertoire involved in the recognition of the representative pathogenic epitope, $VP1_{233\text{-}250}$, appears to be very diverse (Kim et al., 1999): fine epitope regions recognized by individual hybridomas are broad and largely overlapping, but not identical. Although close to 50% of the T cell hybridomas reactive to $VP1_{233\text{-}250}$ used the T cell receptor $V\beta16$, the CDR3 region was extremely heterogeneous among the T cell clones. However, $V\beta16$ (but not $V\alpha$) appears to be associated with recognition of the C-terminal residue of the minimal T cell epitope. Nevertheless, the broad diversity and complexity of the T cell repertoire towards the predominant viral determinants on capsid proteins are apparent despite the limited number of epitope regions involved in T cell recognition.

3. PROTECTIVE ROLE OF $CD8^+$ T CELL RESPONSES

The potential role of $CD8^+$ T cells in the pathogenesis of demyelination has been controversial. A group of investigators proposed that cytotoxic T cells (CTL) specific for virus-infected cells are necessary for clinical manifestation. This is based on the observation that CTL-defective, perforin-deficient C57BL/6 mice do not develop clinical symptoms (Murray et al., 1998; Rivera-Quinones et al., 1998). However, this conclusion could be misleading because these mice are capable of developing clinical symptoms, especially following immunization with UV-inactivated virus (unpublished observation). Moreover, treatment of susceptible mice with anti-CD8 antibodies does not alter the course of TMEV-induced demyelinating disease (Borrow et al., 1992). We and others have shown that viral infection can lead to clinical symptoms even in β_2-microglobulin-deficient resistant mice lacking functional CD8$^+$ T cells (Fiette et al., 1993; Pullen and Kim, 1991). In addition, β_2-microglobulin-deficient susceptible SJL mice also develop demyelinating disease (unpublished observation). These results strongly suggest that virus--specific CTLs are not likely involved in the pathogenesis of demyelination. Recently, it has also been demonstrated that a high level of CTLs is induced in resistant mice and a low level in susceptible mice (Dethlefs et al., 1997). Thus, the inconsistent level of virus-specific CTLs in susceptible SJL mice (Lin et al., 1998; Lindsley et al., 1991) may reflect a poor CD8$^+$ T cell response, indicating a protective role of CD8$^+$ cytotoxic T cells, perhaps by limiting virus-infected cells. Adoptive transfer of CD8$^+$ T cells confers resistance to TMEV-induced demyelination in susceptible recipient mice (Nicholson et al., 1996), again consistent with a protective role of CD8$^+$ CTLs. Therefore, the major role of virus-specific CTLs is most likely for protection rather than tissue damage leading to clinical symptoms.

4. LESSONS LEARNED FROM CYTOKINE MANIPULATION

Several investigators further explored the potential role of proinflammatory cytokines in the virus-induced pathogenesis of demyelination (Table 1). Since bacterial lipopolysaccharide (LPS) produced by Gram negative bacteria and IL-1 are known to potentiate an immune response and trigger the production of various inflammatory cytokines, the effects of LPS or IL-1 on TMEV-induced demyelinating disease were assessed (Pullen et al., 1995). Intraperitoneal injection of LPS or IL-1β into genetically resistant C57BL/6 mice, concomitant with viral infection, resulted in clinical symptoms in approximately 50% of the group compared to 0% in control mice. The increase in susceptibility following LPS-treatment correlated with enhanced levels of TMEV-specific Th1 response as measured by delayed type hypersensitivity and proliferation. Similar LPS treatment of susceptible SJL/J mice, after infection with a low-pathogenic variant of TMEV, resulted in 80–100% of the mice developing clinical symptoms, while none of the control mice were affected clinically (Palma et al., 1996). These results strongly suggest that an increase in the general inflammatory response is capable of promoting a virus-specific Th1 response and inducing demyelinating disease in resistant mice infected with pathogenic virus or susceptible mice infected with a non-pathogenic virus.

Table 1. Effects of cytokines or antibodies to various cytokines on Theiler's murine encephalomyelitis virus-induced demyelinating disease (TMEV-IDD)

Cytokines or antibodies	Effects on TMEV-IDD	References
IL-1/LPS	Induces demyelinating disease in resistant mice	Pullen et al., 1995
	Renders low-pathogenic virus pathogenic	Palma et al., 1996
TNF-α/anti-TNF-α	rTNF-α inhibits the level of demyelination	Paya et al., 1990
	Anti-TNFα inhibits demyelinating disease	Inoue et al., 1996
	Inhibitors for TNF-α suppress development and progression of demyelinating disease	Fushimi et al., 1998; Yamazaki et al., 1997
IL-12/anti-IL-12	Anti-IL-12 inhibits demyelinating disease	Inoue et al., 1998
	Anti-IL-12 does not inhibit demyelination	Bright et al., 1999
IFN-γ/anti-IFN-γ	IFN-γ and anti-IFN-γ exacerbate demyelinating disease	Pullen et al., 1994
	Anti-IFN-γ accelerate demyelination	Rodriguez et al., 1995
	IFN-γ receptor deficiency converts resistant mice to susceptible	Fiette et al., 1995
iNOS	Antagonists inhibit development and progression of demyelinating disease and inflammatory responses	Iwahashi et al., 1999; Rose et al., 1998

iNOS – inducible nitric oxide synthase.

The effects of additional representative cytokines involved in inflammatory responses, such as IFN-γ and TNF-α, have also been investigated. To examine the potential role of IFN-γ, anti-IFN-γ antibody was administered to virus-infected mice (Pullen et al., 1994; Rodriguez et al., 1995). This treatment significantly accelerated the disease course and enhanced Th1 responses towards viral antigens. However, intracerebral injection of recombinant IFN-γ also accelerated the disease similarly (Pullen et al., 1994). Interestingly, virus-induced demyelination was also accelerated in IFN-γ-receptor deficient mice (Fiette et al., 1995). These results suggest that IFN-γ is not necessary for developing demyelination, although its presence can exacerbate the disease. Thus, other proinflammatory cytokines, such as TNF-α, may be able to replace this cytokine function. The potential effects of other proinflammatory cytokines on TMEV-induced demyelination have also been investigated. For example, antibodies to TNF-α or IL-12 (Bright et al., 1999; Fushimi et al., 1998; Inoue et al., 1996; 1998), as well as administration of rIL-4 (unpublished observation), were able to significantly delay the development and reduce the severity of TMEV-induced demyelination. In addition, treatment of susceptible mice with phosphatidylserine or pentoxifylline, which inhibit the production of TNF-α and IFN-γ, significantly reduced the incidence and severity of disease (Fushimi et al., 1998; Yamazaki et al., 1997). These results strongly suggest that the reduction in the proinflammatory cytokine level does provide a beneficial effect on virally induced demyelinating disease. In contrast, Paya et al. (1990) reported that administration of rTNF-α prior to and during viral infection reduced demyelination in the spinal cords. However, these discrepancies may reflect differences in the timing of treatment with respect to viral infection that could be critical for the prevention and/or amelioration of disease (Bright et al., 1999; Inoue et al., 1998). Antibody-mediated reduction in the level of an effector molecule, inducible nitric oxide synthase, acting downstream of these inflammatory cytokines, was also found to be beneficial to the disease (Iwahashi et al., 1999; Rose et al., 1998). These results strongly suggest that proinflammatory cytokines resulting from the Th1 response to the virus are responsible for the pathogenesis of demyelination, as seen with MS (Benvenuto et al., 1992; Correale et al., 1995; Rieckmann et al., 1995).

5. POTENTIAL PATHOGENIC MECHANISMS OF DEMYELINATION

The involvement of virus-specific Th1 responses in the pathogenesis of demyelination is supported by strong experimental data. In addition, the fact that autoimmune responses to the major myelin components are followed by the initial inflammatory response to viral antigens supports the potential involvement of "epitope spreading" in the pathogenesis of demyelination (Miller et al., 1997). The ability of direct lysis of the host cells by this virus may also contribute to the release of autoantigens that can potentially participate in the induction of the autoimmune responses observed later in the disease. The local presentation of viral epitopes to infiltrating $CD4^+$ Th1 lymphocytes in the CNS may also be a critical step for both the initiation and progression of the immune-mediated tissue damage following viral infection (Fig. 2). MHC class II molecules can be expressed on neuroglial cells following exposure to proinflammatory cytokines such as IFN-γ (Wong et al., 1984) or virus particles (Massa et al., 1986). For example, proinflammatory cytokine-activated astrocytes further activate virus-specific $CD4^+$ T cells and, consequently, undergo Fas-mediated apoptosis by the activated T cells *in vivo* as well as *in vitro* (Palma et al., 1999). Since astrocytes play an integral role in maintaining the blood-brain barrier (Eddleston and Mucke, 1993; Montgomery, 1994), such apoptosis of astrocytes most likely contributes to the pathogenesis of TMEV-induced demyelination by compromising the barrier integrity. This is consistent with previous studies suggesting the role of

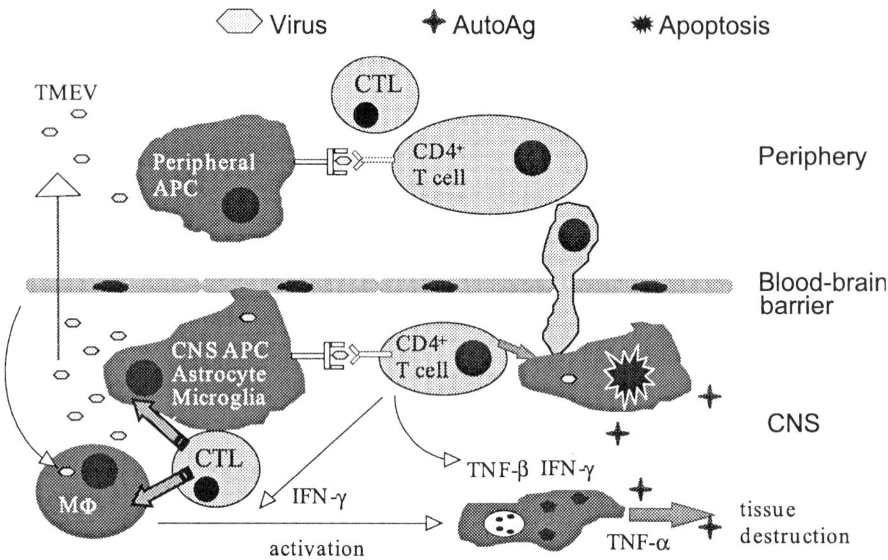

Figure 2. Potential pathogenic mechanisms involved in the immune-mediated demyelination induced following TMEV infection. Resident glial cells may also be activated by inflammatory cytokines and become competent antigen-presenting cells that further stimulate inflammatory Th1 cell response in the CNS. Such T cell activation may consequently lead to breaching the blood brain barrier by cytokines and/or apoptosis of CNS cells. The tissue destruction leads to further release of autoantigens facilitating autoimmunity. Virus-specific CTLs may be involved in the elimination of virus-infected resident CNS cells and macrophages, limiting pathogenic virus-specific Th1 responses

Fas-FasL interaction in MS (Dowling et al., 1996) and, similarly, in autoimmune mouse models of demyelination (Malipiero et al., 1997; Sabelko et al., 1997; Waldner et al., 1997). In addition, activation of astrocytes induces a variety of immunoregulatory cytokines (Lee et al., 1993; Wesselingh et al., 1990), chemokines attracting various inflammatory cells (Tani et al., 1996), as well as adhesion and costimulatory molecules (Nikcevich et al., 1997; Shrikant et al., 1995). Similarly, virus infection itself may also activate a variety of genes, including chemokines, involved in the immune response (unpublished data). Overall, these may promote the influx of inflammatory cells into the CNS and further amplify immune-mediated demyelination. Inhibition of these critical proinflammatory cytokine functions may be sufficient for the significant delay or amelioration of the disease. Therefore, a precise understanding of the pathogenic mechanisms involved in this virus-induced demyelinating disease will provide important general information regarding the initiation and progression of various tissue-specific autoimmune diseases.

Acknowledgment. This work was supported by United States Public Health Service Grants, NS28752, NS33008, and NS23349.

REFERENCES

Adams R. and Victor M. (1977): Principles of neurology. McGraw Hill, New York.

Alvord E. C., Kies M. W. and Suckling A. J. (1984): Experimental allergic encephalomyelitis: a useful model for multiple sclerosis. A. R. Liss, New York.

Benvenuto R., Paroli M., Buttinelli C., Franco A., Barnaba V., Fieschi C. and Balsano F. (1992): Tumor necrosis factor-alpha and interferon-gamma synthesis by cerebrospinal fluid-derived T cell clones in multiple sclerosis. Ann. NY Acad. Sci., **650**, 341–346.

Borrow P., Tonks P., Welsh C. J. and Nash A. A. (1992): The role of $CD8^+$ T cells in the acute and chronic phases of Theiler's murine encephalomyelitis virus-induced disease in mice. J. Gen. Virol., **73**, 1861–1865.

Bright J. J., Rodriguez M. and Sriram S. (1999): Differential influence of interleukin-12 in the pathogenesis of autoimmune and virus-induced central nervous system demyelination. J. Virol., **73**, 1637–1639.

Correale J., Gilmore W., McMillan M., Li S., McCarthy K., Le T. and Weiner L. P. (1995): Patterns of cytokine secretion by autoreactive proteolipid protein-specific T cell clones during the course of multiple sclerosis. J. Immunol., **154**, 2959–2968.

Dal Canto M. C., Kim B. S., Miller S. D. and Melvold R. W. (1996): Theiler's murine encephalomyelitis virus (TMEV)-induced demyelination: a model for human multiple sclerosis. Methods, **10**, 453–461.

Daniels J. B., Pappenheimer A. M. and Richardson S. (1952): Observations on encephalomyelitis of mice (DA strain). J. Exp. Med., **96**, 517–530.

Dethlefs S., Brahic M. and Larsson-Sciard E. L. (1997): An early, abundant cytotoxic T-lymphocyte response against Theiler's virus is critical for preventing viral persistence. J. Virol., **71**, 8875–8878.

Dowling P., Shang G., Raval S., Menonna J., Cook S. and Husar W. (1996): Involvement of the CD95 (APO-1/Fas) receptor/ligand system in multiple sclerosis brain. J. Exp. Med., **184**, 1513–1518.

Eddleston M. and Mucke L. (1993): Molecular profile of reactive astrocytes – implications for their role in neurologic disease. Neuroscience, **54**, 15–36.

Fiette L., Aubert C., Brahic M. and Rossi C. P. (1993): Theiler's virus infection of beta2-microglobulin-deficient mice. J. Virol., **67**, 589–592.

Fiette L., Aubert C., Muller U., Huang S., Aguet M., Brahic M. and Bureau J. F. (1995): Theiler's virus infection of 129Sv mice that lack the interferon alpha/beta or interferon gamma receptors. J. Exp. Med., **181**, 2069–2076.

Fushimi T., Inoue A., Koh C. S., Yamazaki M., Ishihara Y. and Kim B. S. (1998): The effect of pentoxifylline (PTX) on Theiler's murine encephalomyelitis (TMEV)-induced demyelinating disease. Cell. Immunol., **186**, 140–146.

Inoue A., Koh C. S., Yahikozawa H., Yanagisawa N., Yagita H., Ishihara Y. and Kim B. S. (1996): The level of tumor necrosis factor-alpha producing cells in the spinal cord correlates with the degree of Theiler's murine encephalomyelitis virus-induced demyelinating disease. Int. Immunol., **8**, 1001–1008.

Inoue A., Koh C. S., Yamazaki M., Yahikozawa H., Ichikawa M., Yagita H. and Kim B. S. (1998): Suppressive effect on Theiler's murine encephalomyelitis virus-induced demyelinating disease by the administration of anti-IL-12 antibody. J. Immunol., **161**, 5586–5593.

Iwahashi T., Inoue A., Koh C. S., Shin T. K. and Kim B. S. (1999): Expression and potential role of inducible nitric oxide synthase in the central nervous system of Theiler's murine encephalomyelitis virus-induced demyelinating disease. Cell. Immunol., **194**, 186–193.

Johnson R. T. (1975): The possible viral etiology of multiple sclerosis. Adv. Neurol., **13**, 1–46.

Kim B. S., Bahk Y. Y., Kang H. K., Yauch R. L., Kang J. A., Park M. J. and Ponzio N. M. (1999): Diverse fine specificity and receptor repertoire of T cells reactive to the major VP1 epitope (VP1230-250) of Theiler's virus: V beta restriction correlates with T cell recognition of the c-terminal residue. J. Immunol., **162**, 7049–7057.

Kim B. S., Yauch R. L., Bahk Y. Y., Kang J. A., Dal Canto M. C. and Hall C. K. (1998): A spontaneous low-pathogenic variant of Theiler's virus contains an amino acid substitution within the predominant VP1(233-250) T-cell epitope. J. Virol., **72**, 1020–1027.

Lee S. C., Liu W., Dickson D. W., Brosnan C. F. and Berman J. W. (1993): Cytokine production by human fetal microglia and astrocytes. Differential induction by lipopolysaccharide and IL-1 beta. J. Immunol., **150**, 2659–2667.

Lin X., Pease L. R., Murray P. D. and Rodriguez M. (1998): Theiler's virus infection of genetically susceptible mice induces central nervous system-infiltrating CTLs with no apparent viral or major myelin antigenic specificity. J. Immunol., **160**, 5661–5668.

Lindsley M. D., Thiemann R. and Rodriguez M. (1991): Cytotoxic T cells isolated from the central nervous systems of mice infected with Theiler's virus. J. Virol., **65**, 6612–6620.

Lipton H. L. and Friedmann A. (1980): Purification of Theiler's murine encephalomyelitis virus and analysis of the structural virion polypeptides: correlation of the polypeptide profile with virulence. J. Virol., **33**, 1165–1172.

Malipiero U., Frei K., Spanaus K. S., Agresti C., Lassmann H., Hahne M., Tschopp J., Eugster H. P. and Fontana A. (1997): Myelin oligodendrocyte glycoprotein-induced autoimmune encephalomyelitis is chronic/relapsing in perforin knockout mice, but monophasic in Fas- and Fas ligand-deficient lpr and gld mice. Eur. J. Immunol., **27**, 3151–3160.

Massa P. T., Dorries R. and ter Meulen V. (1986): Viral particles induce Ia antigen expression on astrocytes. Nature, **320**, 543–546.

McFarlin D. E. and McFarland H. F. (1982): Multiple sclerosis (first of two parts). N. Engl. J. Med., **307**, 1183–1188.

Miller S. D., Vanderlugt C. L., Begolka W. S., Pao W., Yauch R. L., Neville K. L., Katz-Levy Y., Carrizosa A. and Kim B. S. (1997): Persistent infection with Theiler's virus leads to CNS autoimmunity via epitope spreading. Nat. Med., **3**, 1133–1136.

Montgomery D. L. (1994): Astrocytes: form, functions, and roles in disease. Vet. Pathol., **31**, 145–167.

Murray P. D., McGavern D. B., Lin X., Njenga M. K., Leibowitz J., Pease L. R. and Rodriguez M. (1998): Perforin-dependent neurologic injury in a viral model of multiple sclerosis. J. Neurosci., **18**, 7306–7314.

Nicholson S. M., Dal Canto M. C., Miller S. D. and Melvold R. W. (1996): Adoptively transferred CD8+ T lymphocytes provide protection against TMEV-induced demyelinating disease in BALB/c mice. J. Immunol., **156**, 1276–1283.

Nikcevich K. M., Gordon K. B., Tan L., Hurst S. D., Kroepfl J. F., Gardinier M., Barrett T. A. and Miller S. D. (1997): IFN-gamma-activated primary murine astrocytes express B7 costimulatory molecules and prime naive antigen-specific T cells. J. Immunol., **158**, 614–621.

Palma J. P., Park S. H. and Kim B. S. (1996): Treatment with lipopolysaccharide enhances the pathogenicity of a low-pathogenic variant of Theiler's murine encephalomyelitis virus. J. Neurosci. Res., **45**, 776–785.

Palma J. P., Yauch R. L., Lang S. and Kim B. S. (1999): Potential role of CD4+ T cell-mediated apoptosis of activated astrocytes in Theiler's virus-induced demyelination. J. Immunol., **162**, 6543–6551.

Paya C. V., Leibson P. J., Patick A. K. and Rodriguez M. (1990): Inhibition of Theiler's virus-induced demyelination *in vivo* by tumor necrosis factor alpha. Int. Immunol., **2**, 909–913.

Pullen L. C. and Kim B. S. (1991): Identification of a suitable target cell line for Theiler's murine encephalomyelitis virus specific CTL. FASEB J., **75**, 150.

Pullen L. C., Miller S. D., Dal Canto M. C., Van der Meide P. H. and Kim B. S. (1994): Alteration in the level of interferon-gamma results in acceleration of Theiler's virus-induced demyelinating disease. J. Neuroimmunol., **55**, 143–152.

Pullen L. C., Park S. H., Miller S. D., Dal Canto M. C. and Kim B. S. (1995): Treatment with bacterial LPS renders genetically resistant C57BL/6 mice susceptible to Theiler's virus-induced demyelinating disease. J. Immunol., **155**, 4497–4503.

Rieckmann P., Albrecht M., Kitze B., Weber T., Tumani H., Broocks A., Luer W., Helwig A. and Poser S. (1995): Tumor necrosis factor-alpha messenger RNA expression in patients with relapsing-remitting multiple sclerosis is associated with disease activity. Ann. Neurol., **37**, 82–88.

Rivera-Quinones C., McGavern D., Schmelzer J. D., Hunter S. F., Low P. A. and Rodriguez M. (1998). Absence of neurological deficits following extensive demyelination in a class I-deficient murine model of multiple sclerosis. Nat. Med., **4**, 187–193.

Rodriguez M., Lafuse W. P., Leibowitz J. and David C. S. (1986): Partial suppression of Theiler's virus-induced demyelination *in vivo* by administration of monoclonal antibodies to immune-response gene products (Ia antigens). Neurology, **36**, 964–970.

Rodriguez M., Pavelko K. and Coffman R. L. (1995): Gamma interferon is critical for resistance to Theiler's virus-induced demyelination. J. Virol., **69**, 7286–7290.

Rose J. W., Hill K. E., Wada Y., Kurtz C. I., Tsunoda I., Fujinami R. S. and Cross A. H. (1998): Nitric oxide synthase inhibitor, aminoguanidine, reduces inflammation and demyelination produced by Theiler's virus infection. J. Neuroimmunol., **81**, 82–89.

Sabelko K. A., Kelly K. A., Nahm M. H., Cross A. H. and Russell J. H. (1997): Fas and Fas ligand enhance the pathogenesis of experimental allergic encephalomyelitis, but are not essential for immune privilege in thc central nervous system. J. Immunol., **159**, 3096–3099.

Shrikant P., Weber E., Jilling T. and Benveniste E. N. (1995): Intercellular adhesion molecule-1 gene expression by glial cells. Differential mechanisms of inhibition by IL-10 and IL-6. J. Immunol., **155**, 1489–1501.

Soldan S. S., Berti R., Salem N., Secchiero P., Flamand L., Calabresi P. A., Brennan M. B., Maloni H. W., McFarland H. F., Lin H. C., Patnaik M. and Jacobson S. (1997): Association of human herpes virus 6 (HHV-6) with multiple sclerosis: increased IgM response to HHV-6 early antigen and detection of serum HHV-6 DNA. Nat. Med., **3**, 1394–1397.

Tani M., Glabinski A. R., Tuohy V. K., Stoler M. H., Estes M. L. and Ransohoff R. M. (1996): *In situ* hybridization analysis of glial fibrillary acidic protein mRNA reveals evidence of biphasic astrocyte activation during acute experimental autoimmune encephalomyelitis. Am. J. Pathol., **148**, 889-896.

Theiler M. and Gard S. (1940): Encephalomyelitis of mice. J. Exp. Med., **72**, 49–67.

Waldner H., Sobel R. A., Howard E. and Kuchroo V. K. (1997): Fas- and FasL-deficient mice are resistant to induction of autoimmune encephalomyelitis. J. Immunol., **159**, 3100–3103.

Welsh C. J., Tonks P., Nash A. A. and Blakemore W. F. (1987): The effect of L3T4 T cell depletion on the pathogenesis of Theiler's murine encephalomyelitis virus infection in CBA mice. J. Gen. Virol., **68**, 1659–1667.

Wesselingh S. L., Gough N. M., Finlay-Jones J. J. and Mc Donald P. J. (1990): Detection of cytokine mRNA in astrocyte cultures using the polymerase chain reaction. Lymphokine Res., **9**, 177–185.

Wong G. H., Bartlett P. F., Clark-Lewis I., Battye F. and Schrader J. W. (1984): Inducible expression of H-2 and Ia antigens on brain cells. Nature, **310**, 688–691.

Yahikozawa H., Inoue A., Koh C. S., Choe Y. K. and Kim B. S. (1997): Major linear antibody epitopes and capsid proteins differentially induce protective immunity against Theiler's virus--induced demyelinating disease. J. Virol., **71**, 3105–3113.

Yamazaki M., Inoue A., Koh C. S., Sakai T. and Ishihara Y. (1997): Phosphatidylserine suppresses Theiler's murine encephalomyelitis virus-induced demyelinating disease. J. Neuroimmunol., **75**, 113–122.

Yauch R. L., Kerekes K., Saujani K. and Kim B. S. (1995): Identification of a major T-cell epitope within VP3 amino acid residues 24 to 37 of Theiler's virus in demyelination-susceptible SJL/J mice. J. Virol., **69**, 7315–7318.

Yauch R. L. and Kim B. S. (1994): A predominant viral epitope recognized by T cells from the periphery and demyelinating lesions of SJL/J mice infected with Theiler's virus is located within VP1(233-244). J. Immunol., **153**, 4508–4519.

Yauch R. Y., Palma J. P., Yahikozawa H., Koh C.-S. and Kim B. S. (1998): Role of individual T cell epitopes of Theiler's virus in the pathogenesis of demyelination correlates with the ability to induce a Th1 response. J. Virol., **72**, 6169–6174.

EVIDENCE THAT FAS AND FASL CONTRIBUTE TO THE PATHOGENESIS OF EXPERIMENTAL AUTOIMMUNE ENCEPHALOMYELITIS

BONNIE N. DITTEL

Blood Research Institute, Blood Center of Southeastern Wisconsin, Milwaukee, WI 53201-2178, USA

Abstract The well established and characterized animal model for the human demyelinating autoimmune disease multiple sclerosis (MS) is known as experimental autoimmune encephalomyelitis (EAE) (Olsson, 1995). EAE is clinically characterized by focal areas of inflammation and demyelination and an infiltrate composed of large numbers of lymphocytes and macrophages, often found in a perivascular localization but also throughout the central nervous system (CNS) (Martin and McFarland, 1995). Active immunization of mice with several different protein components of myelin, including myelin basic protein (MBP), proteolipid protein (PLP) and myelin oligodendrocyte glycoprotein (MOG), are capable of eliciting an immune response resulting in the quintessential symptoms of EAE: ascending paralysis involving the tail and then the limbs. Depending on the mouse strain and myelin antigen utilized, the disease course can be acute or chronic relapsing, characterized by a rapid onset of hind limb weakness that commonly progresses to paralysis, followed by spontaneous remission starting 7–10 days after the initial appearance of symptoms. EAE can also be induced passively by the adoptive transfer of *in vitro* activated $CD4^+$ T cell clones or lines, typically of the Th1 phenotype, into irradiated susceptible recipients (Baron et al., 1993). The mechanisms involved in the cellular pathogenesis leading to paralysis and demyelination have been extensively studied and are primarily mediated by $CD4^+$ T cells of the Th1 phenotype, with specificity for myelin antigens. Following activation, Th1 CD4 T cells produce in abundance the inflammatory cytokines TNF-α, IFN-γ and lymphotoxin α (LT-α, also know as TNF-β). IFN-γ production is highly correlated with encephalitogenicity and may contribute to disease by up-regulation of adhesion molecules on endothelial cells, facilitating migration of lymphocytes into the CNS; by induction of major histocompatibility complex (MHC) class I and MHC class II molecules on astrocytes, microglial cells and brain endothelium, facilitating antigen (Ag) presentation in the CNS; and by activation of macrophages, leading to production of nitric oxide, a potent cytotoxic molecule. TNF-α and LT-α are both members of the TNF family of molecules and cause cell death by apoptosis following interaction with their counter-receptors, the TNFR1 and TNFR2, leading to a cascade of proteolytic

A. Górski et al. (eds.), Autoimmunity, 95–108.

events culminating in the blebbing of the cytoplasmic membrane, nuclear condensation and DNA fragmentation (Clement and Stamenkovic, 1994; Nagata and Suda, 1995). Consequently, the production of TNF-α and LT-α by Th1 clones has been correlated with encephalitogenic potential (Powell et al., 1990) and antibodies (Abs) to both prevents EAE upon transfer of encephalitogenic clones (Ruddle et al., 1990). Even though substantial evidence exists for the role of inflammatory cytokines in the pathogenesis of EAE, other mechanisms of myelin destruction are thought to exist. To date, many reports have implicated a role for the cell death-inducing ligand pair Fas and Fas-ligand (FasL).

Key words: Fas; Fas ligand; experimental autoimmune encephalomyelitis.

1. FAS AND FASL IN CD4+ T CELL-MEDIATED CELLULAR CYTOTOXICITY

In addition to effector functions of $CD4^+$ T cells mediated through the production of cytokines, $CD4^+$ T cells also have the capacity to mediate the cytotoxicity of appropriate targets. This cytotoxicity was recently shown to be primarily mediated by the interaction of Fas on the target cell with the FasL on the $CD4^+$ T cell, leading to the apoptotic cell death of the Fas-expressing cell (Ashany, 1995; Hahn et al., 1995a; Hanabuchi et al., 1994; Henkart, 1994; Lynch et al., 1995). Fas (APO-1, CD95) is a member of the TNF-receptor superfamily (Itoh et al., 1991) and was first identified with the use of a monoclonal antibody (mAb), which induced apoptosis upon binding to some tumor cells (Trauth et al., 1989; Yonehara et al., 1989). FasL has also recently been cloned and is a type II membrane protein with homology to members of the TNF family (Suda et al., 1993). Resting $CD4^+$ T cells do not express FasL on the cell surface, but activation either by antigen (peptide/MHC class II) or nonspecifically with anti-CD3, ConA or PMA/ionomycin leads to the rapid appearance of cell surface FasL (El-Khatib et al., 1995; Hahn et al., 1995a; 1995b; Hanabuchi et al., 1994; Suda et al., 1995). Using Th1, Th2 and Th0 clones bearing identical T cell receptors (TCR) (Dittel et al., 1997), we were able to demonstrate up-regulation of FasL following stimulation with PMA/ionomycin on all three types of Th clones (Fig. 1). Our findings are consistent with other reports demonstrating that some Th2 clones can express FasL (Fig. 1) (Hahn et al., 1995a; 1995b; Suda et al., 1995). Although cytotoxicity mediated by Fas/FasL is primarily a function of Th1 and Th0 cells, several reports have described killing by Th2 cells (Lancki et al., 1991; Suda et al., 1995). Utilizing the same Th0, Th1 and Th2 clones, we demonstrate antigen-specific killing of a target cell by all three clones (Fig. 2). At least one

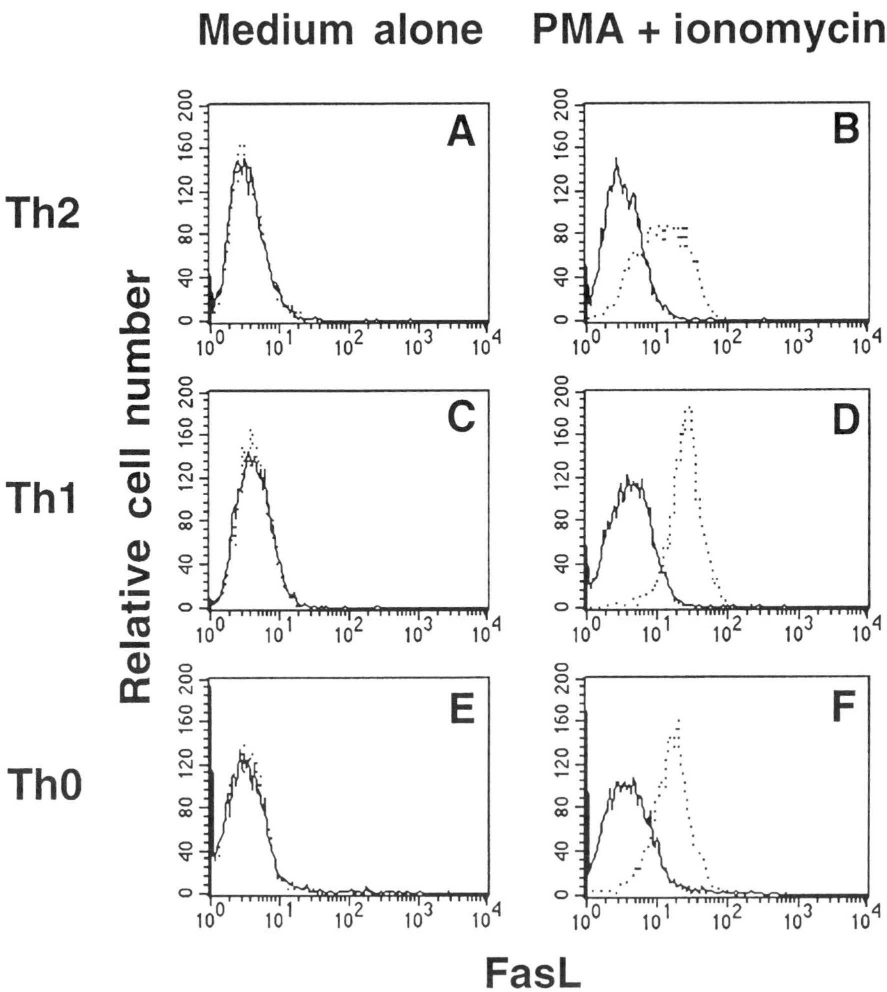

Figure 1. Expression of FasL after activation with PMA/ionomycin and antigen stimulation. Expression of cell surface FasL was analyzed by a three-step indirect immunofluorescence staining and flow cytometry. The D10. TCR Th2 (A, B), Th1 (C, D) and Th0 (E, F) clones were incubated with anti-FasL (10 μg/ml) (PharMingen, San Diego, CA) followed by a second incubation with anti-mouse IgG-biotin and concluded with a third incubation with strepavidin-PE. Antibody incubations were carried out on ice with two washes following each step and the cells were fixed in 1% paraformaldehyde and analyzed using CellQuest on a FACScan® (Becton Dickinson, Mountain View, CA). Negative controls consisted of cells incubated with anti-mouse IgG-biotin followed by strepavidin-PE. Expression of the FasL was measured after a 6-hour incubation at 37°C with medium alone or in the presence of PMA (10 ng/ml) and ionomycin (1 mM) in six-well microtiter plates. Histograms represent fluorescence intensity on the horizontal axis and relative cell number on the vertical axis. The background staining is depicted in each histogram as a solid line and FasL specific staining is shown as a dotted line

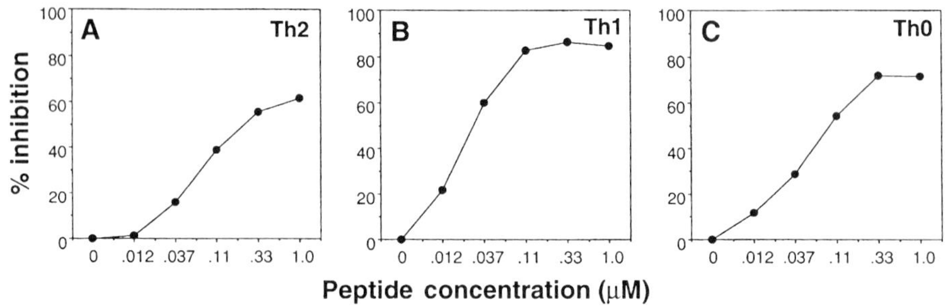

Figure 2. Antigen specific cytotoxicity by the D10. TCR Th2, Th1 and Th0 clones stimulated with the antigenic peptide CA134-146 from the antigen hen egg conalbumin to which the D10. TCR is restricted in the context of I-A^k. Mitomycin-c inactivated D10. TCR clones were cocultured with CH27 cells (I-A^k) in the presence of 1:3 dilutions of CA134-146 from 0.012 to 1 μM. After 16–18 h the cultures were pulsed with 1 μCi [^{3}H] TdR and harvested after an additional 4 h of incubation. Data for the Th2 clone is shown in A, for the Th1 clone in B and for the Th0 clone in C. Data is presented as % inhibition of CH27 growth calculated as follows: (1 – CPM in presence of peptide: CPM in absence of peptide) × 100

report has shown that Th2 cells can be encephalitogenic under specific conditions (Lafaille et al., 1997). Thus, although EAE is primarily thought to be a consequence of pathogenicity mediated by Th1 cells, the role for Th2 cells either in pathogenicity, or in protection/recovery due to production of Th2 cytokines, such as IL-4 and IL-10, has yet to be firmly established (Cua et al., 1995; Falcone and Bloom, 1997).

The potential importance for Fas/FasL-mediated cell death in the regulation of homeostasis within the immune system is demonstrated by dysregulation of T cell populations leading to lymphadenopathy, splenomegaly and autoimmune disorders (Lynch et al., 1995; Nagata and Suda, 1995). In addition to T cells killing target cells in an antigen-specific manner, several reports have shown that activated Th1 cells expressing FasL can lyse Fas-expressing targets in the absence of TCR ligation (El-Khatib et al., 1995; Hahn et al., 1995b; Suda et al., 1995). This nonspecific killing has been shown by several groups to include fratricidal T cell killing (Hahn et al., 1995b; Su et al., 1993) and T cell suicide (Brunner et al., 1995; Dhein et al., 1995; Hahn et al., 1995b; Lynch et al., 1995). Since Fas is expressed by both Th1 and Th2 cells (Fig. 3), self-reactive T cell populations in EAE could potentially be controlled either in the periphery or in the CNS by promoting death of Th1 or Th2 cells following up-regulation of FasL, leading to cell death by fratricide and/or suicide.

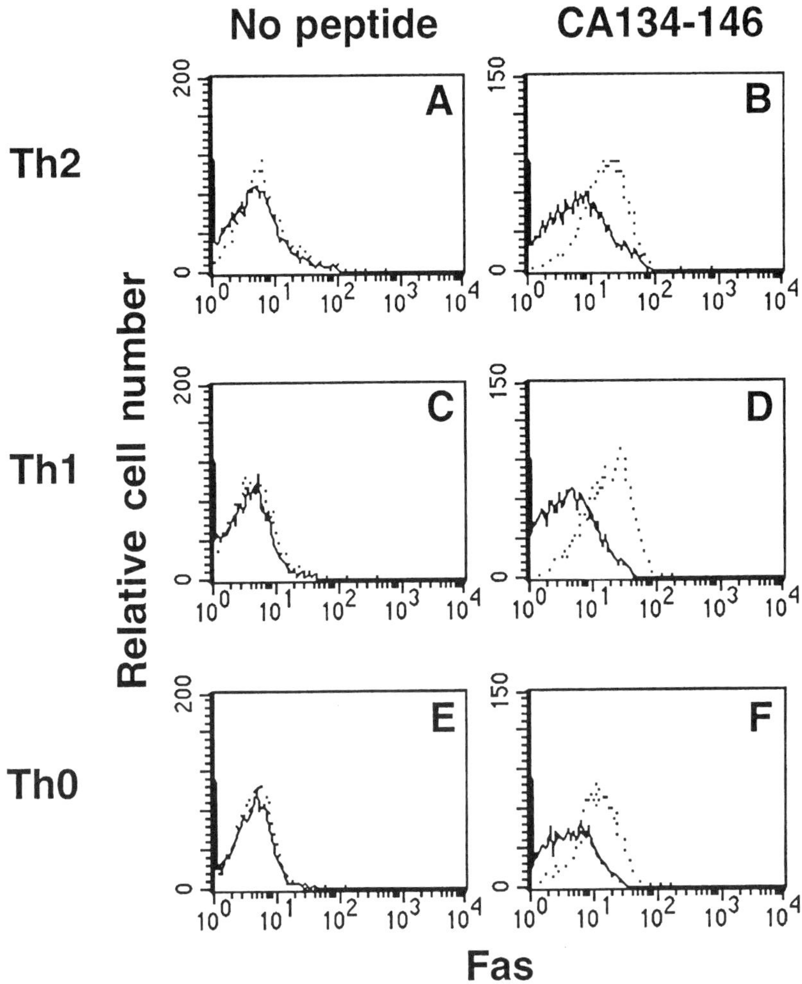

Figure 3. Up-regulation of cell surface Fas following antigen stimulation. The D10. TCR Th2 (A, B), Th1 (C, D) and Th0 (E, F) clones were stimulated with 100 μM CA 134-146 (second column) or with medium alone (first column) using B10.BR spleen cells as APC. After 48 h, Fas was detected by direct immunofluorescence with anti-mouse Fas-PE (PharMingen, San Diego, CA). Histograms represent fluorescence intensity on the horizontal axis and relative cell number on the vertical axis. The background staining is depicted in each histogram as a solid line and Fas specific staining is shown as a dotted line

2. FAS EXPRESSION IN THE CNS IS IMPORTANT FOR THE DEVELOPMENT OF EAE

The role of Fas/FasL interactions in EAE have been facilitated by the presence of mice carrying autosomal recessive mutations in the genes encoding Fas (lpr) and FasL (gld) (Nagata and Suda, 1995). Fas is disrupted in lpr mice by an endogenous retrovirus insertion carrying a poly(A) adenylation signal on the long terminal repeats, leading to truncation of the mRNA (Nagata and Suda, 1995). In gld mice, the gene encoding FasL has a point mutation in the cytoplasmic region of the protein that disrupts interaction with Fas (Nagata and Suda, 1995). Several independent reports suggested a role for the cell death-inducing molecules Fas and FasL in the pathogenesis of EAE (Malipiero et al., 1997; Sabelko et al., 1997; Waldner et al., 1997). In these studies, mice deficient in Fas or FasL were immunized with myelin antigens and assessed for clinical signs of EAE. The study by Sabelko et al. (1997) utilized guinea pig (gp) MBP-immunized B10.PL-lpr mice and showed almost complete protection from the paralytic clinical symptoms of EAE. Of interest was the similar T cell infiltrate observed in the spinal cords of Fas-deficient mice and wild-type (wt) mice, suggesting that Fas and FasL do not contribute to the process of T cell migration into the CNS. Several groups investigated active EAE induction using MOG35-55 in C57BL/6 mice carrying the lpr or gld mutations with contrasting results. Waldner et al. (1997) reported almost complete protection for EAE in both B6-gld and B6-lpr mice, with wt mice exhibiting a relapsing-remitting disease course. Similarly, a report by Okuda et al. (1998) also showed protection in C57BL/6-lpr mice immunized with MOG35-55. In contrast, the study performed by Malipiero et al. (1997) showed only partial protection in disease severity, with lpr and gld mice exhibiting a monophasic disease course and the wt mice exhibiting a chronic disease course. The discrepancies in these two studies may be reflected by the more aggressive disease induction protocol employed by the Malipiero group, using a higher concentration of pertussis toxin and boosting with Ag 1 week following primary Ag challenge. The protection reported by the Waldner group may partially reflect disease induced in older male mice that are less susceptible to disease than female mice.

The relative role of Fas/FasL in the pathogenesis of EAE seems to be affected either by the antigen used or by the strain of mouse the experiments are being carried out on, or both. This is evident from a recent study by Suvannavejh et al. (2000) in which EAE induced in SJL mice deficient in Fas following active immunization with a peptide from PLP resulted in chronic progressive disease of greater severity as compared to the relapsing-remitting disease course observed in their heterozygote littermates. Although no differences were observed in the acute phase of disease, the chronic disease in the SJL-lpr mice was accompanied by an increase in mononuclear cells infiltrating the spinal cord (Suvannavejh et al., 2000). These data suggest that Fas/FasL play a role in recovery from EAE in the SJL mouse, presumably by eliminating the self-reactive T cell population in the CNS.

The active induction of EAE in gld or lpr mice as performed in the above studies does not definitively reveal the cell populations in which the presence of Fas and FasL are important in EAE. To test whether Fas and FasL expression are important on the T cell or in the CNS, we performed adoptive transfer experiments to passively induce EAE, targeting the deficiency in Fas and FasL to the transferred T cells, the recipient or both (Dittel et al., 1999). These experiments revealed that B10.PL-lpr mice deficient in Fas were protected against EAE induction following adoptive transfer of an activated Th1 T cell line generated from a TCR transgenic mouse specific for a peptide of MBP comprised of the first 11 amino acids (Ac1-11). In comparison, B10.PL mice adoptively transferred with the same T cell line succumbed to disease with symptoms appearing around day 8 and peaking around day 15 with an acute monophasic disease course characterized by hind limb paresis and paralysis (Dittel et al., 1999). Recovery from disease symptoms was observed around day 24 following T cell transfer (Dittel et al., 1999). We attribute the protection observed in the Fas deficient recipients to a blockage of Fas-induced cell death because of the absence of functional Fas expression in the CNS. This conclusion is supported by the reverse experiment, showing no disease protection when Fas-deficient T cells are transferred into wt recipients. Thus, protection was only observed when Fas was deficient in the CNS. The role for Fas expression in the CNS in EAE was also demonstrated by Sabelko-Downes et al. (1999) using similar adoptive transfer procedures.

Surprisingly, we saw no protection when Fas-deficient T cells were transferred into Fas-deficient recipients (Dittel et al., 1999). We attribute this result to the loss of homeostatic regulation of the transferred T cell population by Fas and FasL (Singer et al., 1994). Thus, the absence of Fas on the transferred T cell population may disrupt cell death of the activated T cells, allowing the T cells to accumulate in sufficient numbers to cause EAE by a mechanism that is clearly unrelated to Fas/FasL. To examine the possibility that the lack of protection is due to accumulation of the Fas-deficient T cells, we measured the percentage of transgenic T cells in the $CD4^+$ T cell population in the spleens and lymph nodes 7 and 14 days following adoptive transfer (Table 1). On day 7 following transfer of wt T cells into Fas-deficient recipients, 26% of the splenic $CD4^+$ T cell population were transgenic. This number was reduced to 16% when the T cells were transferred into an lpr recipient. These data suggest that the transferred T cell population is elimi-

Table 1. Percentage of CD4+ cells that express the MBP TCR transgene in the spleen and lymph nodes of B10.PL and B10.PL-1pr mice adoptively transferred with MBP-wt or MBP-lpr T cells

Adoptive transfer[a]	Day 7		Day 14	
	spleen (%)	lymph node[b] (%)	spleen (%)	lymph node (%)
MBP-wt into B10.PL	26[c]	52	31	25
MBP-wt into lpr	16	35	28	26
MBP-lpr into B10.PL	81	83	37	37
MBP-lpr into lpr	83	92	40	43

[a] 1×10^6 CD4+ T cells isolated from MBP TCR transgenic mice with or without the lpr mutation were i. v. transferred into irradiated (600 rads) B10.PL or B10.PL-lpr mice 4 days following antigen specific activation.

[b] Lymph node cells include cells from the popliteal, auxiliary and inguinal lymph nodes.

[c] The percentage of total CD4+ T cells isolated from the spleen or lymph nodes of B10.PL or B10.PL-lpr recipient mice that express the MBP TCR as assessed by staining with a mAb specific for Vβ8.2, the TCRβ chain expressed by the MBP TCR.

nated in the periphery, perhaps by host Fas-deficient lymphocytes, which have been reported to express enhanced levels of FasL (Chu et al., 1995). In contrast, the transfer of Fas-deficient T cells into either wt or lpr mice resulted in elevated numbers of transgenic T cells, with more than 80% of the CD4+ splenocytes being of donor origin (Table 1). As shown in Table 1, similar results were observed in lymph node CD4 T cell populations. Interestingly, on day 14 the percentage of transgenic T cells in the mice that received wt T cells increased, while the mice transferred with lpr T cells had reduced numbers of transgenic T cells. Overall, these data suggest that the lack of protection following transfer of lpr T cells into lpr recipients may partially be due to the accumulation of T cells in the periphery, generating a greater pool of T cells with encephalitogenic potential.

Interestingly, in the study by Sabelko-Downes et al. (1999), protection from EAE was observed when lpr T cells were transferred into lpr recipients. This group also examined preferential elimination of transferred wt T cells into lpr recipients and saw no difference as compared to controls on days 3 and 5 (Sabelko-Downes et al., 1999). However, to conduct this analysis the authors used allogeneic T cells and did not assess the levels of Fas on the cell surface of the transferred T cell population. The discrepancy between our study and that of Sabelko-Downes et al. (1999) could be attributed to the differences in generation of the T cell lines. In our study, the T cells were fully differentiated Th1 effector cells, having been rested for 7–10 days before reactivation and transfer (Dittel et al., 1999). In the Sabelko-Downes et al. (1999) study, the T cells were stimulated with antigen for 4 days before transfer with no rest. This activation protocol may have been too short in duration to allow differentiation of the naïve T cells into polarized Th1 effectors cells. In addition, the authors did not analyze the cytokine profiles of the transferred cells. In our study, we showed that the transferred T cell populations expressed high levels of the Th1 inflammatory cytokines IFN-γ, TNF-α and LT-α and low levels of the Th2 cytokines IL-4, IL-5 and IL-10 (Dittel et al., 1999). If high levels of IL-4 and IL-10 were produced by the transferred T cell population in the Sabelko-Downes et al. (1999) study, this could have contributed to protection, as both these cytokines have been implicated in protection from EAE.

3. FASL EXPRESSION ON THE ENCEPHALITOGENIC T CELL POPULATION IS IMPORTANT IN THE REGULATION OF EAE

We also examined the role of FasL in the CNS and on the transferred T cell population. In agreement with Sabelko-Downes et al. (1999), we found that the expression of FasL on the transferred T cell population is important for the development of EAE. This was demonstrated by protection from EAE when FasL was deficient on the transferred T cells (Dittel et al., 1999; Sabelko-Downes et al., 1999), while no protection was observed when wt T cells were transferred into gld recipients, of interest is the enhanced disease observed under these experimental conditions (Dittel et al., 1999; Sabelko-Downes et al., 1999). We observed this enhancement as an earlier onset of disease and a longer, more severe disease course, suggesting that FasL expression in the recipient animal is involved in the regulation of the encephalitogenic T cell population (Dittel et al., 1999). This hypothesis was more fully examined by Sabelko-Downes et al. (1999), who also observed more severe EAE of longer duration in gld recipients by examining spinal cord infiltrates in wt and gld mice. Infiltrates during the early/acute phase of disease (day 23) were similar in the two groups of mice (Sabelko-Downes et al., 1999). However, differences were observed during the late/chronic stage of disease, with diminished infiltration in wt mice as compared to clusters of $CD4^+$ cells observed in the gld recipients (Sabelko-Downes et al., 1999). The observation of groups of T cells remaining late after transfer suggests that the FasL deficient host is unable to effectively eliminate the infiltrating encephalitogenic T cells.

Although Fas/FasL have been shown to be involved in the pathogenesis of

EAE, no role for either molecule has been demonstrated in the migration of T cells into the CNS. This was demonstrated following active induction of EAE in lpr mice where disease was suppressed, but the infiltration observed into the CNS 10 days following immunization was comparable to wt mice (Sabelko et al., 1997). However, reduced levels of apoptotic cells were observed in the lesions of the lpr mice, again suggesting a role for Fas in the apoptosis of cells in the CNS. The cells undergoing apoptosis in the CNS have yet to be definitively identified, but a logical target cell would be the myelin-producing oligodendrocyte. Fas expression has been generally demonstrated in the CNS in patients with MS (Dowling et al., 1996) and specifically on the oligodendrocyte population (D'Souza et al., 1996).

4. CONCLUSION

The evidence accumulating from multiple laboratories using different mouse strains, thus utilizing different myelin antigens, has clearly demonstrated a role for Fas/Fas ligand not only in the pathogenesis of EAE in the CNS, but in the regulation of the encephalitogenic T cell population as well. In keeping with the subtle differences in the data from various laboratories, a mechanism for the role of Fas and FasL in EAE is shown in Fig. 4. As shown in Fig. 4, the early pathogenesis in the CNS is most likely mediated by a small number of $CD4^+$ T cells that express FasL. We found that the adoptive transfer of a large number of T cells could circumvent the protection observed in Fas-deficient mice (Wong et al., 1999). FasL expressed by activated T cells infiltrating the CNS would interact with Fas on oligodendrocytes, presumably up-regulated by IFN-γ (Nagata and Golstein, 1995; Nagata and Suda, 1995) produced by the Th1 encephalitogenic T cells, leading to apoptotic death of oligodendrocytes. This early cell destruction would then lead to a full inflammatory response and the recruitment of additional autoreactive T cells, macrophages and other cell types to the site of immune attack, forming an inflammatory lesion. The ensuing myelin destruction would provide ample Ag for the continued activation and expansion of the autoreactive T cell pool. As the autoreactive Th1 cells accumulate, the local production of the pathogenic Th1 cytokines, IFN-γ, TNF-α and LT-α, would also increase, resulting in continued apoptotic death of oligodendrocytes and demyelination. Macrophages in the lesion may contribute to oligodendrocyte destruction by the production of nitric oxide (Bogdan, 1998). The escalating inflammatory response could then be dampened by any number of proposed mechanisms, including T cell apoptosis by Fas/FasL and the emergence of a Th2 response (O'Garra et al., 1997).

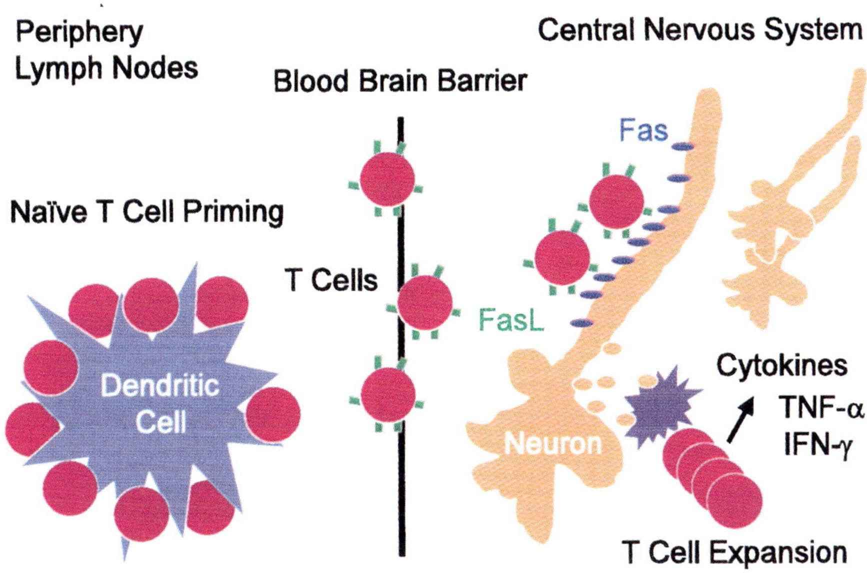

Figure 4. Model for the role of Fas and FasL in the pathogenesis of EAE in the CNS. Priming of naïve CD4+ T cells (light purple) with self-antigen in the peripheral lymph nodes by dendritic cells as antigen-presenting cells results in activated Th1 T cells expressing FasL (green) with the capacity to migrate across the blood-brain barrier. The first self-antigen-specific T cells to enter the CNS secrete inflammatory cytokines, up-regulating adhesion molecules and MHC class II molecules on endothelium and resident microglial cells in the CNS and potentially Fas (blue) on oligodendrocytes. The self-antigen-specific T cells expressing FasL interact with Fas expressed by oligodendrocytes that form a layer of myelin (orange) around the neuronal axon, causing cell death of the oligodendrocytes. Myelin antigens released following the apoptotic death of oligodendrocytes are taken up by antigen-presenting cells (possibly microglia), processed and presented to the infiltrating T cells. The T cells are reactivated, resulting in renewed proliferation leading to an expansion of Th1 T cells, allowing for local accumulation of the Th1 cytokines (TNF-α, IFN-γ and LT-α) at high levels. This local accumulation of cytokine production leads to a full-blown inflammatory response and could also result in further apoptotic cell death of oligodendrocytes through the TNFRs

REFERENCES

Ashany D., Song X., Lacy E., Nikolic-Zugic J., Friedman S. M. and Elkon K. B. (1995): Th1 CD4+ lymphocytes delete activated macrophages through the Fas/APO-1 antigen pathway. Proc. Natl. Acad. Sci. USA, **92**, 11225–11229.

Baron J. L., Madri J. A., Ruddle N. H., Hashim G. and Janeway C. A. Jr. (1993): Surface expression of α4 integrin by CD4 T cells is required for their entry into brain parenchyma. J. Exp. Med., **177**, 57–68.

Bogdan C. (1998): The multiplex function of nitric oxide in (auto)immunity. J. Exp. Med., **187**, 1361–1365.

Brunner T., Mogil R. J., La Face D., Yoo N. J., Mahboubi A., Echeverri F., Martin S. J., Force W. R., Lynch D. H., Ware C. F. and Green D. R. (1995): Cell-autonomous Fas (CD95)/Fas--ligand interaction mediates activation-induced apoptosis in T-cell hybridomas. Nature, **373**, 441–444.

Clement M.-V. and Stamenkovic I. (1994): Fas and tumor necrosis factor receptor-mediated cell death: similarities and distinctions. J. Exp. Med., **180**, 557–567.

Chu J. L., Ramos P., Rosendorff A., Nikolic-Zugic J., Lacy E., Matsuzawa A. and Eldon K. B. (1995): Massive upregulation of the Fas ligand in lpr and gld mice: implications for Fas regulation and the graft-versus-host disease-like wasting syndrome. J. Exp. Med., **181**, 393–398.

Cua D. J., Hinton D. R. and Stohlman S. A. (1995): Self-antigen-induced Th2 responses in experimental allergic encephalomyelitis (EAE)-resistant mice. Th2-mediated suppression of autoimmune disease. J. Immunol., **155**, 4052–4059.

Dhein J., Walczak H., Baumler C., Debatin K.-M. and Krammer P. H. (1995): Autocrine T-cell suicide mediated by APO-1/(FAS/CD95). Nature, **373**, 438–441.

Dittel B. N., Merchant R. M. and Janeway C. A. Jr. (1999): Evidence for Fas-dependent and Fas-independent mechanisms in the pathogenesis of experimental autoimmune encephalomyelitis. J. Immunol., **162**, 6392–6400.

Dittel B. N., Sant' Angelo D. B. and Janeway C. A. Jr. (1997): Peptide antagonists inhibit proliferation and the production of IL-4 and/or IFN-gamma in T helper 1, T helper 2, and T helper 0 clones bearing the same TCR. J. Immunol., **158**, 4065–4073.

Dowling P., Shang G., Raval S., Menonna J., Cook S. and Husar W. (1996): Involvement of the CD95 (APO-1/Fas) receptor/ligand system in multiple sclerosis brain. J. Exp. Med., **184**, 1513–1518.

D'Souza S. D., Bonetti B., Balasingam K. B., Cashman N. R., Barker P. A., Troutt A. B., Raine C. S. and Antel J. P. (1996): Multiple sclerosis: Fas signaling in oligodendrocyte cell death. J. Exp. Med., **184**, 2361–2370.

El-Khatib M., Stanger B. Z., Dogan H., Cui H. and Ju S.-T. (1995): The molecular mechanism of FasL-mediated cytotoxicity by $CD4^+$ Th1 clones. Cell. Immunol., **163**, 237–244.

Falcone M. and Bloom B. R. (1997): A T helper cell 2 (Th2) immune response against non-self antigens modifies the cytokine profile of autoimmune T cells and protects against experimental allergic encephalomyelitis. J. Exp. Med., **185**, 901–907.

Hahn S., Gehri R. and Erb P. (1995a): Mechanism and biological significance of CD4-mediated cytotoxicity. Immunol. Rev., **146**, 57–79.

Hahn S., Stalder T., Wernli M., Burgin D., Tschopp J., Nagata S. and Erb P. (1995b): Down-modulation of $CD4^+$ T helper type 2 and type 0 cells by T helper type 1 cells via Fas/Fas-ligand interaction. Eur. J. Immunol., **25**, 2679–2685.

Hanabuchi S., Koyanagi M., Kawasaki A., Shinohara N., Matsuzawa A., Nishimura Y., Kobayashi Y., Yonehara S., Yagita H. and Okumura K. (1994): Fas and its ligand in a general mechanism of T-cell-mediate cytotoxicity. Proc. Natl. Acad. Sci. USA, **91**, 4930–4934.

Henkart P. A. (1994): Lymphocyte-mediated cytotoxicity: Two pathways and multiple effector molecules. Immunity, **1**, 343–346.

Itoh N., Yonehara S., Ishii A., Yonehara M., Mizushima S., Sameshima M., Hase A., Seto Y. and Nagata S. (1991): The polypeptide encoded by the cDNA for human cell surface antigen Fas can mediate apoptosis. Cell, **66**, 223–243.

Lafaille J. J., van de Keere F., Hsu A. L., Baron J. L., Haas W., Raine C. S. and Tonegawa S. (1997): Myelin basic protein-specific T helper 2 (Th2) cells cause experimental autoimmune encephalomyelitis in immunodeficient hosts rather than protect them from the disease. J. Exp. Med., **186**, 307–312.

Lancki D. W., Hsieh C. S. and Fitch F. W. (1991): Mechanisms of lysis by cytotoxic T lymphocyte clones. Lytic activity and gene expression in cloned antigen-specific $CD4^+$ and $CD8^+$ T lymphocytes. J. Immunol., **146**, 3242–3249.

Lynch D. H., Ramsdell F. and Alderson M. R. (1995): Fas and FasL in the homeostatic regulation of immune responses. Immunol. Today, **16**, 569–574.

Malipiero U., Frei K., Spanaus K.-S., Agresti C., Lassmann H., Hahne M., Tschopp J., Eugster H.-P. and Fontana A. (1997): Myelin oligodendrocyte glycoprotein-induced autoimmune encephalomyelitis is chronic/relapsing in perforin knockout mice, but monophasic in Fas- and Fas ligand-deficient lpr and gld mice. Eur. J. Immunol., **27**, 3151–3160.

Martin R. and McFarland H. F. (1995): Immunological aspects of experimental allergic encephalomyelitis and multiple sclerosis. Crit. Rev. Clin. Lab. Sci., **32**, 121–182.

Nagata S. and Golstein P. (1995): The Fas death factor. Science, **267**, 1449–1456.

Nagata S. and Suda T. (1995): Fas and Fas ligand: lpr and gld mutations. Immunol. Today, **16**, 39–43.

O'Garra A., Steinman L. and Gijbels K. (1997): $CD4^+$ T-cell subsets in autoimmunity. Curr. Opin. Immunol., **9**, 872–883.

Okuda Y., Bernard C. C. A., Fujimura H., Yanagihara T. and Sakoda S. (1998): Fas has a crucial role in the progression of experimental autoimmune encephalomyelitis. Mol. Immumol., **35**, 317–326.

Olsson T. (1995): Critical influences of the cytokine orchestration or the outcome of myelin antigen-specific autoimmunity in experimental autoimmune encephalomyelitis and multiple sclerosis. Immunol. Rev., **144**, 245–268.

Powell M. B., Mitchell D., Lederman J., Buckmeier J., Zamvil S. S., Graham M., Ruddle N. H. and Steinman L. (1990): Lymphotoxin and tumor necrosis factor-α production by myelin basic protein-specific T cell clones correlates with encephalitogenicity. Int. Immunol., **2**, 539–554.

Ruddle N. H., Bergman C. M., McGrath K. M., Lingenheld E. G., Grunnet M. L., Padula S. J. and Clark R. B. (1990): An antibody to lymphotoxin and tumor necrosis factor prevents transfer of experimental allergic encephalomyelitis. J. Exp. Med., **172**, 1193–1200.

Sabelko K. A., Kelly K. A., Nahm M. H., Cross A. H. and Russell J. H. (1997): Fas and Fas ligand enhance the pathogenesis of experimental allergic encephalomyelitis, but are not essential for immune privilege in the central nervous system. J. Immunol., **159**, 3096–3099.

Sabelko-Downes K. A., Cross A. H. and Russell J. H. (1999): Dual role for Fas ligand in the initiation of and recovery from experimental allergic encephalomyelitis. J. Exp. Med., **189**, 1195–1205.

Singer G. G., Carrera A. C., Marshak-Rothstein A., Martínez C. and Abbas A. K. (1994): Apoptosis, Fas and systemic autoimmunity: the MRL-lpr/lpr model. Curr. Opin. Immunol., **6**, 913–920.

Su M. W.-C., Walden P. R. and Eisen H. N. (1993): Peptide-induced destruction of CD8+ cytotoxic T lymphocytes is due to fratricide. J. Immunol., **151**, 658–667.

Suda T., Okazaki T., Naito Y., Yokota T., Arai N., Ozaki S., Nakao K. and Nagata S. (1995): Expression of the Fas ligand in cells of T cell lineage. J. Immunol., **154**, 3806–3813.

Suda T., Takahashi T., Golstein P. and Nagata S. (1993): Molecular cloning and expression of the Fas ligand, a novel member of the tumor necrosis factor family. Cell, **75**, 1169–1178.

Suvannavejh G. C., Dal Canto M. C., Matis L. A. and Miller S. D. (2000): Fas-mediated apoptosis in clinical remissions of relapsing experimental autoimmune encephalomyelitis. J. Clin. Invest., **105**, 223–231.

Trauth B. C., Klas C., Peters A. M. J., Matzku S., Moller P., Flak W., Debatin K. M. and Krammer P. H. (1989): Monoclonal antibody-mediated tumor regression by induction of apoptosis. Science, **245**, 301–305.

Waldner H., Sobel R. A., Howard E. and Kuchroo V. K. (1997): Fas- and FasL-deficient mice are resistant to induction of autoimmune encephalomyelitis. J. Immunol., **159**, 3100–3103.

Wong F. S., Dittel B. N. and Janeway C. A. Jr. (1999): Transgenes and knockout mutations in animal models of type 1 diabetes and multiple sclerosis. Immunol. Rev., **169**, 93–100.

Yonehara S., Ishii A. and Yonehara M. (1989): A cell-killing monoclonal antibody (anti-fas) to a cell surface antigen co-downregulated with the receptor of tumor necrosis factor. J. Exp. Med., **169**, 1747–1756.

THE ROLE OF CYTOKINES IN EXPERIMENTAL AUTOIMMUNE ENCEPHALOMYELITIS

ESTELLE BETTELLI and LINDSAY B. NICHOLSON

Center for Neurologic Diseases, Brigham and Women's Hospital and Harvard Medical School, Boston MA 02115, USA

Abstract Experimental autoimmune encephalomyelitis (EAE) is an animal model of the demyelinating disease multiple sclerosis. In EAE cytokines play a critical role in defining the Th1 or Th2 nature of the autoantigen directed immune response, and in propagating and regulating inflammation within the central nervous system. In this review we summarize some of the recent developments in the field of cytokine research that relate to this model of human disease, focusing principally on disease induced with the autoantigens myelin proteolipid protein and myelin oligodendrocyte protein.

Key words: experimental autoimmune encephalomyelitis; cytokines; proteolipid protein; myelin oligodenodrocyte protein; review.

1. INTRODUCTION

The immune system depends on a complex interplay between many specialized cell types for the effective control of infection. These interactions are mediated both by cell surface receptors, and by the secretion of soluble protein mediators, especially cytokines. Cytokines fall into several overlapping categories: growth factors, such as interleukin2 (IL-2) or IL-7; general mediators of inflammation, such as IL-1 and IL-6; and cytokines associated with the differentiation and regulation of subsets of $CD4^+$ (and also $CD8^+$) T lymphocytes. In autoimmune diseases such as multiple sclerosis (MS), where an aberrant immune response to self proteins leads to inflammation and the destruction of normal tissue, the role of cytokines has been intensively studied, often with conflicting or contradictory results. In this review we will summarize recent work in the area of inflammatory autoimmune disease of the central nervous system (CNS) in the animal model of MS, experimental autoimmune encephalomyelitis (EAE) (Alvord et al., 1984).

A. Górski et al. (eds.), Autoimmunity, 109–127.

EAE in mice is a complex process that may be induced by immunization with a pathogenic CNS-derived protein or peptide (usually given in conjunction with pertussis toxin or vaccine), or by the transfer of autoantigen-specific T cells into unimmunized recipients (Sobel et al., 1994; Wekerle, 1993), or it may arise spontaneously in mice transgenic for T cell receptors (TCRs) which recognize myelin antigens (Goverman et al., 1993; Lafaille et al., 1994; Waldner et al., 2000). Many proteins that cause disease have been identified. We have been particularly interested in EAE caused by peptides derived from myelin proteolipid protein (PLP), amino acids 139-151 and 178-191 (Nicholson et al., 1997a) in IA^s mice and from myelin oligodendrocyte protein (MOG), amino acids 35-55, which causes disease in IA^b mice (Bettelli et al., 1998). The other very well-known encephalitogenic protein is myelin basic protein (MBP), which causes disease in IA^u mice (Zamvil and Steinman, 1990). Several further candidate encephalitogenic proteins have been identified in recent years (Waksman, 1995).

Clinical EAE is usually a relapsing/remitting disease in mice. It is useful to consider the disease as having an induction phase, which occurs in the periphery following immunization, and an effector phase, which occurs in the CNS where activated T cells encounter myelin antigens in their natural state. These phases are subject to normal, but poorly understood, immunoregulatory effects which are likely to be, in part, cytokine mediated, but with costimulatory molecules such as CD80/86 and CD40/CD40L also playing a crucial role (Chang et al., 1999; Grewal et al., 1996; Kuchroo et al., 1995).

Cytokines from all categories have been shown to be important in the disease process. The T lymphocyte phenotype, which has a crucial impact on the outcome of a number of infectious disease models (Mosmann and Sad, 1996; Reiner et al., 1993; Romagnani, 1994), is particularly important. The description of CNS autoantigen-specific T helper type 1 (Th1) cells, which secrete interferon γ (IFN-γ) and lymphotoxin α (LT-α), also known as tumor necrosis factor β (TNF-β), and T helper type 2 (Th2) cells which secrete IL-4, IL-5, IL-10 and IL-13, has stimulated a great deal of investigation in EAE. Analysis of the phenotype of T cell clones specific for a number of different CNS autoantigens has shown quite clearly that in immuno-competent animals pathogenic cells are of the Th1 phenotype (Nicholson and Kuchroo, 1996; Zamvil and Steinman, 1990). The role of Th2 cells is more controversial. Cells of this phenotype can be protective (Kuchroo et al., 1995), but they may have no effect on disease and in immuno-compromised animals they may be pathogenic, inducing a histologically atypical form of EAE (Lafaille et al., 1997). Th3 cells, which secrete transforming growth factor β (TGF-β), regulate EAE and can protect animals from disease (Chen et al., 1994). Therefore, T cells of different phenotypes appear to have different and somewhat complimentary roles in EAE. However, the mechanisms by which T cells differentiate into these different phenotypes *in vivo* is not well understood. Several factors are known to regulate this process, including the cytokines present at priming (especially IL-4 and IL-12), the concentration and nature of the antigen and the modulation of costimulatory molecules, but the relative importance of these and other factors is not clear (Nicholson et al., 1997b).

Most studies of cytokines in EAE have sought to address the role of specific cytokines in the disease process. Three experimental approaches have been predominantly used: the systemic administration of cytokine or blocking antibodies, over-expression of the cytokine of interest by transgenesis, sometimes in an organ- or cell-specific fashion, and targeted disruption of specific cytokine genes to produce gene-knockout mice. It has been something of a surprise to learn from many of these studies, and with different cytokines, that the effects anticipated from the paradigm that Th1 cytokines cause disease and Th2 cytokines protect from disease are not always borne out in experiments. These findings can be explained in several non-exclusive ways. The Th1/Th2 paradigm may be a poor predictor of outcome in the case of autoimmune disease (Lafaille, 1998); the effects on autoimmune disease of cytokine redundancy in mice deficient in a particular cytokine from birth may be fundamentally different from those of cytokine deficiency in an acute disease setting (Steinman, 1997); the interpretation of studies with blocking antibodies is difficult *in vivo* because of questions as to whether antibodies are stimulatory or blocking and whether they have variable penetration into different organs; and specific cytokines which are associated with pathogenic cells may be crucial for inducing regulatory mechanisms. These hypotheses need further experimental clarification.

2. CYTOKINES ASSOCIATED WITH THE TH1 PHENOTYPE

2.1. IL-12 and IL-18

IL-12 is a heterodimeric cytokine of 70 kDa (p70) composed of two covalently linked chains, p40 and p35. Transcript of the p35 gene is constitutively expressed in most cell types. However, the p35 chain is secreted efficiently only when it is associated with the p40 chain forming a heterodimer. p40 transcripts are expressed only in cells capable of producing active IL-12. Most IL-12 is produced by monocytes/macrophages in response to bacterial products and intracellular parasites. However, both B cells and murine dendritic cells can also produce some IL-12 (Trinchieri and Scott, 1995).

IL-12 promotes the differentiation of naïve T cells into Th1 cells (Hsieh et al., 1993; Seder et al., 1993) and induces high levels of IFN-γ production by Th1 cells and NK cells. IL-12 enhances IgG2a, IgG2b and IgG3 isotype antibody production (complement-fixing isotypes associated with Th1 responses) and, on the other hand, inhibits IgG1 isotype antibody production, which is associated with Th2 responses. IL-12 has also been shown to enhance the lytic activity of NK cells and to enhance cytotoxic T lymphocyte (CTL) responses. IL-12 and IFN-γ can act together in a positive feedback loop which enhances the generation of Th1 cells.

In EAE, RT-PCR analysis has shown that IL-12 p40 mRNA is elevated in the brain and the lymphoid organs of animals in the acute phase of disease (Issazadeh et al., 1995). Administration of IL-12 to SJL/J mice increases disease severity (Leonard et al., 1996), and treatment of animals with anti-IL12 antibody was able to attenuate EAE in animals receiving MBP reactive cells or PLP reactive cells (Leonard et al., 1995). In a recent study (Segal et al., 1998), C57Bl/6 IL-12$^{-/-}$ mice were found to be resistant to EAE induced by MBP. In this study, the authors showed that IL-12 was essential for the pathogenesis of EAE, in contrast to effector molecules such as IFN-γ, which may be redundant, since IFN-γ$^{-/-}$ mice which were highly susceptible to disease could be protected from EAE by anti-IL-12 antibody treatment.

IL-18 (previously known as IFN-γ-inducing factor IGIF) works in synergy with IL-12 (Ahn et al., 1997). In human systems it has been shown to enhance Th1 differentiation (Micallef et al., 1996) and, in experiments using murine cells, IL-18 and IL-1α had reciprocal effects on Th1 and Th2 cells which were mediated in part by their actions on NF-κB p50/p65 (Robinson et al., 1997). In rats, neutralizing antibodies for IL-18 inhibited the development of EAE, and splenic T cells from treated rats showed changes in the ratio of IL-4: IFN-γ following activation compared with control animals (Wildbaum et al., 1998).

2.2. IFN-γ and TNF-α

The roles of IFN-γ and TNF in EAE and MS have been investigated intensively. In early studies, the presence of both cytokines was shown to correlate with disease and, because of their pro-inflammatory nature (TNF-α) and association with Th1 T cell differentiation (IFN-γ), they have been the subject of many studies to discover the utility of targeted therapeutic intervention. The surprising finding which emerges from these studies in mice is that they are not required for disease to develop and that their absence can promote, rather than prevent, disease.

IFN-γ is secreted by activated T cells and macrophages and has many reported functions including promoting T cell growth and inhibiting IL-4--mediated B cell growth and murine IgG1 and IgE secretion. IFN-γ up-regulates class II MHC molecules, adhesion molecules and activates macrophages. Its secretion is also the hallmark of Th1-type T cells and, on this basis, it was rational to predict that inhibiting IFN-γ would ameliorate EAE. This prediction has been contested by a number of experiments. Blocking studies with antibody against IFN-γ have often been shown not to reduce disease, but also to exacerbate it (Billiau et al., 1988; Duong et al., 1992). In studies of mice in which IFN-γ or its receptor had been knocked out, these animals were as susceptible or more susceptible to EAE than their littermate controls (Krakowski and Owens, 1996; Zhang et al., 1997). On the other hand, in humans, a clinical trial of systemic IFN-γ exacerbated multiple sclerosis (Panitch and Bever, 1993).

These results might be explained in two ways. First that the secretion of IFN-γ may be necessary to establish the conditions which subsequently regulate the progress of inflammation, and in its absence, because the inflammatory process continues for longer, more tissue damage results. Secondly, the administration of IFN-γ and its inhibitors may have different effects depending upon whether treatment is given in the induction or effector phase. These proposals are the subject of ongoing investigations.

The role of TNF is even more complex and confusing. Two members of the TNF family have been studied intensively in EAE: TNF-α and lymphotoxin (LT-α, TNF-β). TNF-α is secreted by many cell types, including activated T cells, macrophages, microglia and astrocytes. LT-α is produced primarily by T cells and is usually regarded as a Th1 cytokine. There are two known receptors for these cytokines, TNFR1 and TNFR2, which bind TNF-α and LT-α with almost identical affinities. TNF-α/LT-α secretion has been associated with clinical disease and with T cell pathogenicity (Begolka et al., 1998; Kennedy et al., 1992), and in some experiments treatment with antibodies that block the actions of these cytokines reduces disease (Korner et al., 1997a; Ruddle et al., 1990; Selmaj et al., 1991).

Animals with deletions of TNF-α and LT-α genes have been generated. Their analysis has been complicated by the fact that these genes are closely linked to the MHC and, therefore, the MHC haplotype remains that of the strain in which the knockout was made. Within these limitations, it is clear that neither TNF-α nor LT-α are required for the development of EAE and in some experiments its deletion exacerbates disease (Liu et al., 1998) although this is not the case in all systems (Frei et al., 1997; Korner et al., 1997; Suen et al., 1997). Preliminary data from mice in which the TNFR1 (p55) has been disrupted indicate that these mice are resistant to EAE and that this resistance is dependent on the expression of the TNFR1 in the host but not on autoantigen-specific T cells (Willenborg et al., 1998). Anti-TNF-α has been used to treat MS patients and it was found that the patients suffered relapses following treatment (The Lenercept Multiple Sclerosis Study Group, 1999; van Oosten et al., 1996).

Therefore, the elimination of either of these Th1 cytokines by gene targeting does not prevent EAE, demonstrating that individual Th1 cytokines, which are associated with disease-causing cells, are not themselves necessary to cause disease. These studies raise the interesting possibility that the presence of Th1 cytokines is required for normal regulatory processes which subsequently limit tissue damage.

3. GROWTH FACTORS AND INFLAMMATORY CYTOKINES

3.1. IL-1, IL-2, IL-3 and IL-15

IL-1 comprises two cytokines with limited homology but which both bind the same receptor with approximately equivalent affinity. It has an important role in the regulation of inflammatory responses triggered by an innate immune response. IL-1 was originally described as a "costimulator" of T cells and its addition to MBP-specific T cells leads to an exacerbation of clinical disease (Mannie, 1987). In rats, the administration of IL-1 and soluble IL-1R, respectively, exacerbate and ameliorate clinical disease scores (Jacobs et al., 1991).

IL-2 was the first T cell growth factor to be identified and has been studied intensively (Smith, 1988). Systemic treatment with antibodies specific for the rat IL-2 receptor inhibited EAE when the disease was induced by the transfer of autoantigen-specific T cell lines, but not when it was induced by active immunization (Engelhardt et al., 1989). This finding can be explained as a non-specific growth-promoting effect. In mice which have been genetically modified, those with an IL-2 transgene show growth retardation and premature death, and IL-2 knockout mice develop generalized autoimmune disease, especially inflammatory bowel disease and hemolytic anemia (Kroemer et al., 1991; Sadlack et al., 1995; 1993). This condition relates at least in part to a failure of normal T cell homeostasis, specifically a failure of activation-induced cell death (Van Parijs and Abbas, 1998). Therefore, IL-2 can regulate the development of generalized autoimmune disease. Strong evidence for the importance of IL-2 in the development of organ-specific autoimmune disease comes from genetic studies in EAE and diabetes. Genome scans for loci associated with disease have identified a common region on mouse chromosome 3 associated with both diabetes and EAE. Using congenic non-obese diabetic (NOD) mice, the associated locus has recently been narrowed to a 0.15 cM interval encoding *Il2* and *Fgf2*, and a polymorphism shared by the susceptible SJL and NOD mouse strains has been identified in the IL-2 gene (Encinas et al., 1999). However, the mechanism by which this predisposes to autoimmune disease has yet to be clarified.

IL-3 is released from activated T cells but functions mainly as a growth factor for hematopoietic stem cells. It has been over-expressed in the brains of mice by transgenic technology using the GFAP promoter (Chiang et al., 1996; Powell et al., 1999). These mice exhibit macrophage/microglial-mediated primary demyelination, which demonstrates the potential toxicity of this cytokine within the brain. The clinical phenotype of these mice differs from EAE in that the disease is chronic progressive rather that relapsing/remitting however, these studies provide some insight into the potential neurotoxicity of high levels of cytokine within the CNS, which may arise in the vicinity of active inflammation.

IL-15 is a cytokine which binds the β and γ chains of the IL-2R and has some biological effects which resemble those of IL-2 (Waldmann and Tagaya, 1999). It has been associated with Th1 and Th2 differentiation (Ruckert et al., 1998) and is produced in human fetal astrocytes and microglia in response to IL-1-β, IFN-γ and TNF-α. In multiple sclerosis, IL-15 mRNA expression has been correlated with clinical disease in the CNS of patients (Kivisakk et al., 1998).

3.2. IL-6

IL-6 is produced by activated T cells upon antigen stimulation. It is also produced by B cells, macrophages, endothelial cells and fibroblasts (Taga and Kishimoto, 1997). Several studies have implied that IL-6 may play a role in the pathogenicity of EAE. An elevation of IL-6 gene expression in the brain seems to correlate with the severity of the disease (Diab et al., 1997; Kennedy et al., 1992; Okuda et al., 1995). In one report, anti-IL-6 antibody administration has been shown to prevent EAE (Gijbels et al., 1995). However, another report showed that anti-IL-6 injections had no significant effect on disease development and that infection of mice with a vaccinia virus producing recombinant IL-6 could inhibit demyelinating disease (Willenborg et al.,

1995). In a viral model of EAE, IL-6 administration was able to suppress demyelination induced by Theiler's murine encephalomyelitis virus infection (Rodriguez et al., 1994), raising the possibility of a protective role for IL-6 in the development of EAE. However, IL-$6^{-/-}$ mice, generated independently by different groups, are resistant to the development of EAE (Mendel et al., 1998; Okuda et al., 1998; Samoilova et al., 1998b). A small decrease in recombinant MOG-specific T cell proliferation was observed in IL-$6^{-/-}$ mice compared with control mice, and MOG 35-55 specific T cells derived from IL-$6^{-/-}$ mice were unable to transfer disease to a wild-type (wt) recipient, suggesting that, in the absence of IL-6, the generation of pathogenic T cells is impaired *in vivo*. This hypothesis is also supported by the fact that MOG 35--55-specific T cells derived from wt mice induce disease on transfer into IL-$6^{-/-}$ mice. Although a lower anti-MOG antibody response was also observed in IL-$6^{-/-}$ mice, this seems to reflect a generally lower production of antibody in IL-$6^{-/-}$ mice and probably does not explain the resistance to EAE of these mice. The above results suggest a role for IL-6 in the induction of disease and/or as a factor necessary for the pathogenicity of T cells.

4. CYTOKINES ASSOCIATED WITH DISEASE REGULATION

4.1. IL-4 and IL-10

The production of IL-4 is tightly regulated. It is only produced by the Th2 subset of activated T cells, mast cells, NK cells and basophils. IL-4 was initially described as a B cell growth factor (Howard et al., 1982). IL-4 also regulates Ig isotype switching in B cells, stimulating the production of IgG1 and IgE (Kuhn et al., 1991). But one of the main effects of this cytokine on T cells is to drive their differentiation towards the Th2 phenotype (Sedder et al., 1992; Swain et al., 1990). In EAE induced in the SJL mouse strain, several groups have shown increases in IL-4 mRNA expression in the CNS of animals in recovery (Merrill et al., 1992), and PLP-specific-IL-4-producing Th2 clones have been shown to inhibit EAE when they were given at the time of immunization, or to reverse the disease when given at the first signs of EAE (Kuchroo et al., 1995). Direct administration of IL-4 has also been shown in most cases to reduce the severity of EAE (Racke et al., 1994). The use of a T cell hybridoma transduced to express IL-4 has also been shown to ameliorate MBP-induced EAE in (PL/JxSJL/J)F1 mice, although the transfer of hybridoma may cause some other side effects (Shaw et al., 1997).

Examining IL-$4^{-/-}$ mice, Liblau et al. (1997) found that on the PL/J background they developed disease similarly to wt mice, while we and others found that IL-$4^{-/-}$ mice (on the C57Bl/6 background) developed an exacerbated disease (Betteli et al., 1998). Therefore, the absence of IL-4 probably does increase EAE; however, the disease developed by the IL-$4^{-/-}$ mice was much less severe than the disease that developed in IL-$10^{-/-}$ mice. Conversely, while IL-10 transgenic mice were resistant to EAE induction, IL-4 transgenic mice developed a disease similar to their genetically matched littermates. Together, these results suggest that IL-4 may play a role in limiting EAE development, perhaps especially during the disease induction phase, but its role may not be as critical as that of IL-10. A recent study showed that prolonged treatment with IL-10 inhibited EAE development in SJL mice, while IL-4 was ineffective. Moreover, when IL-10 and IL-4 were injected together, IL-4 seemed to abrogate the inhibitory effect of IL-10 (Nagelkerken et al., 1997).

In the mouse system, IL-10 is produced by Th2 and Th0 $CD4^+$ T cells clones, but not by Th1 or $CD8^+$ T cells, although it has been reported that some $CD4^+$ T cells can secrete both IL-10 and IFN-γ (Pohl-Koppe et al., 1998). Recently, a new subset of T cells, Tr1 cells, has been described which produced high levels of IL-10 almost exclusively (Groux et al., 1997). The production of IL-10 by T cells is induced by stimulation with antigen or polyclonal activators, and mouse B cells (especially the Ly1 B cell subset) also produce IL-10 after stimulation, but the major source of IL-10 seems to be macrophages. High production of IL-10 by macrophages occurs upon activation, e.g. by LPS and CNS-resident astrocytes and microglia are also capable of producing IL-10.

IL-10 has been shown to inhibit the synthesis of other cytokines by macrophages, especially pro-inflammatory cytokines such as TNF-α, IL-1 and IL-12, but the production of IL-10 itself by macrophages can also be inhibited in the presence of IL-10. In addition, IL-10 also inhibits expression of MHC class II antigens. Th1 cells are inhibited by IL-10, although this effect appears to be mediated to a large extent via inhibition of IL-12 synthesis by APCs. The role of IL-10 in the differentiation of T cells from naive precursor cells is less clear. In one study, IL-10 was shown to act like IL-4 in the generation of Th2 cells (Hsieh et al., 1992), but in another experiment, IL-10 and anti-IL-10 antibody had little effect on the differentiation into Th2 cells (Romani et al., 1992).

IL-10 mRNA has repeatedly been shown to peak before or during the onset of remission in EAE (Issazadeh et al., 1995; Kennedy et al., 1992) although a recent report showed an almost constant expression of IL-10 mRNA in the brains of animals with EAE (Begolka et al., 1993). Conflicting results have been obtained when recombinant IL-10 or anti-IL-10 antibody were injected *in vivo*. While Rott et al. (1994) found that administration of IL-10 during the induction phase of EAE in rats could suppress the clinical signs of the disease, Cannella et al. (1996) showed that injection of IL-10 in mice worsened its clinical course. When an encephalitogenic PLP 139-151-specific T cell clone transfected with IL-10 was injected into animals, the onset of EAE could be inhibited (Mathisen et al., 1997).

We and others (Betteli et al., 1998; Samoilova et al., 1998a), using MOG 35-55 as the encephalitogenic antigen, have reported that IL-$10^{-/-}$ mice on the C57Bl/6 background develop more severe clinical EAE than wt mice. While analyzing the mechanism by which IL-$10^{-/-}$ mice develop such a severe disease, we found that T cells from these mice exhibit a stronger MOG 35-55-specific proliferation, produce more pro-inflammatory cytokines (IFN-γ and TNF-α) and induce very severe EAE upon transfer into wt mice. One explanation for these findings comes from the work of Segal et al. (1998), who have shown that there is an immunoregulatory circuit between IL-12 and IL-10. Treatment with anti-IL-12 antibody significantly decreases EAE and is associated with an increase in IL-10 production. All these results together strongly suggest that IL-10 may protect from the development of EAE and they highlight the importance of the interplay between inflammatory and regulatory cytokines.

4.2. TGF-β

There are three isoforms of TGF-β, named TGF-β1, TGF-β2 and TGF-β3 (Derynck, 1994). TGF-β is first synthesized as a proprotein which is cleaved by a protease to generate the mature cytokine. Many different cell types, including lymphocytes and macrophages, produce TGF-β. TGF-β has been shown to inhibit proliferation of T and B lymphocytes (Kehrl et al., 1986) and to inhibit the effect or the production of IFN-γ, TNF-α, TNF-β and IL-2 (Espevik et al., 1987). The cytokine exhibits a dual role on monocytes/ /macrophages. TGF-β has a chemotactic effect and induces the expression of inflammatory mediators, such as IL-1 and TNF-α, by monocytes. On the other hand, TGF-β exerts a deactivating effect once the monocytes are differentiated into macrophages, e.g. suppressing peroxide release by these cells (Tsunawaki et al., 1988). TGF-β mRNA in the CNS has been reported to correlate with remission of EAE in the rat model (Issazedeh et al., 1996; Tanuma et al., 1997). Treatment with anti-TGF-β antibody exacerbated clinical signs of EAE (Johns et al., 1991; Kuruvilla et al., 1991; Racke et al., 1992), while administration of TGF-β reduced the severity of disease in animals

(Kuruvilla et al., 1991; Racke et al., 1991). The important role of TGF-β in the regulation of EAE has also been demonstrated in animals made tolerant by feeding them myelin antigens. The oral administration of MBP in rats or in mice suppresses EAE, and TGF-β has an essential role in this protection (Chen et al., 1994; Khoury et al., 1992). Feeding MBP to mice gives rise to regulatory cells, called Th3, cells, which release TGF-β and are able to protect animals from actively induced EAE (Chen et al., 1994; Inobe et al., 1996; Miller et al., 1992). Moreover, T cells producing TGF-β appeared in rats which had spontaneously recovered from disease and they seemed to inhibit IFN-γ production by encephalitogenic T cells, suggesting that TGF-β may exert a direct down-regulatory role on pathogenic T cells (Racke et al., 1991). As well as this direct effect, TGF-β also decreases MHC class II expression on astrocytes, which may limit antigen presentation in the CNS (Schluesener, 1990), and it may also prevent the accumulation of T cells in the CNS by acting on the cerebrovascular endothelium (Santambrogio et al., 1993).

5. CONCLUSIONS

Although it has been shown that the induction of Th1 cells plays a critical role in the development of EAE, the specific role of the cytokines which define this subset of T cells, IFN-γ and TNF-α, remains contradictory. It is possible that, as the immune response progresses, IFN-γ is critical to the induction of regulatory mechanisms that limit the amount of clinical disease and, therefore, that the same cytokine may have opposite effects in the induction and effector phase of disease. The effects of Th2 cytokines with anti-inflammatory properties seem more consistent and, overall, the data indicate an immunomodulatory role for IL-4, IL-10 and TGF-β, although T cells of a Th2 phenotype do not always protect from disease, and in immuno-compromised mice may induce atypical neuroinflammation (Lafaille et al., 1997). These Th2 cytokines may have relatively more or less important roles depending on the specific model in question. Another interesting possibility is that Th1 and Th2 cytokines are markers for pathogenic and protective subsets but are not sufficient, in the absence of other factors, to determine disease phenotype (Nicholson et al., 1998).

It is also clear that genetic background can have a profound influence on the outcome of EAE, and so the analysis of cytokines in different mouse strains, which develop different forms of EAE, further complicates the comparison of different studies. Progress in understanding the role of cytokines in EAE will depend on techniques that allow the simultaneous analysis of several cytokines in the same mouse strain, immunized with the same antigen. Because cytokines can also have different effects depending on the target cell, it is difficult to predict the function of individual cytokines in a complex tissue such as the CNS based on studies carried out *in vitro*. Moreover, *in vivo*, during the priming phase and the effector phase of the disease, the same cytokines may be involved in different positive and negative feedback loops involving multiple cell types. Therefore, a complete understanding of the role of specific cytokines in the disease process will also require a better understanding of how the interplay between the different cytokines and different cells changes as the inflammatory response progresses.

Acknowledgment. Dr. Lindsay B. Nicholson is supported by a grant from the National Institutes of Health (K08 AI01557-01).

REFERENCES

Ahn H. J., Maruo S., Tomura M., Mu J., Hamaoka T., Nakanishi K., Clark S., Kurimoto M., Okamura H. and Fujiwara H. (1997): A mechanism underlyind synergy between IL-12 and IFN-gamma-inducing factor in enhanced production of IFN-gamma. J. Immunol., **159**, 2125–2131.

Alvord E. C., Kies M. W. and Suckling A. J. (1984): Experimental allergic encephalomyelitis: A useful model for multiple sclerosis. Liss, New York.

Begolka W. S., Vanderlug C. L., Rahbe S. M. and Miller S. D. (1998): Differential expression of inflammatory cytokines parallels progression of central nervous system pathology in two clinically distinct models of multiple sclerosis. J. Immunol., **161**, 4437–4446.

Bettelli E., Das M. P., Howard E. D., Weiner H. L., Sobel R. A. and Kuchroo V. K. (1998): IL-10 is critical in the regulation of autoimmune encephalomyelitis as demonstrated by studies of IL-10 and IL-4-deficient and transgenic mice. J. Immunol., **161**, 3299–3306.

Billiau A., Heremans H., Vandekerckhove F., Dijkmans R., Sobis H., Meulepas E. and Carton H. (1988): Enhancement of experimental allergic encephalomyelitis in mice by antibodies against IFN-gamma. J. Immunol., **140**, 1506–1510.

Cannella B., Gao Y. L., Brosnan C. and Raine C. S. (1996): IL-10 fails to abrogate experimental autoimmune encephalomyelitis. J. Neurosci. Res., **45**, 735–746.

Chang T. T., Jabs C., Sobel R. A., Kuchroo V. K. and Sharpe A. H. (1999): Studies in B7-deficient mice reveal a critical role for B7 costimulation in both induction and effector phases of experimental autoimmune encephalomyelitis. J. Exp. Med., **190**, 733–740.

Chen Y., Kuchroo V. K., Inobe J., Hafler D. A. and Weiner H. L. (1994): Regulatory T cell clones induced by oral tolerance: Suppression of autoimmune encephalomyelitis. Science, **265**, 1237–1240.

Chiang C. S., Powell H. C., Gold L. H., Samimi A. and Campbell I. L. (1996): Macrophage/

/microglial-mediated primary demyelination and motor disease induced by the central nervous system production of interleukin-3 in transgenic mice. J. Clin. Invest., **97**, 1512–1524.

Derynck R. (1994): Transforming growth factor-beta. In Thomson A. W. (ed.): The cytokine handbook. Academic Press Ldt, London, 319–342.

Diab A., Zhu J., Xiao B. G., Mustafa M. and Link H. (1997): High IL-6 and low IL-10 in the central nervous system are associated with protracted relapsing EAE in DA rats. J. Neuropathol. Exp. Neurol., **56**, 641–650.

Duong T. T., St. Louis J., Gilbert J. J., Finkelman F. D. and Strejan G. H. (1992): Effect of anti--interferon-gamma and anti-interleukin-2 monoclonal antibody treatment on the development of actively and passibely induced experimental allergic encephalomyelitis in the SJL/J mouse. J. Neuroimmunol., **36**, 105–115.

Encinas J. A., Wicker L. S., Peterson L. B., Mukasa A., Teuscher C., Sobel R., Weiner H. L., Seidman C. E., Seidman J. G. and Kuchroo V. K. (1999): QTL influence autoimmune diabetes and encephalomyelitis map to a 0.15-cM region containing Il2 (letter). Nat. Genet., **21**, 158–160.

Engelhardt B., Diamanstein T. and Werkerle H. (1989): Immunotherapy of experimental autoimmune encephalomyelitis (EAE): Differential effect of anti-IL-2 receptor antibody therapy on actively induced and T-line mediated EAE in the Lewis rat. J. Autoimmun., **2**, 61–73.

Espevik T., Figari I. S., Shalaby M. R., Lackides G. A., Lewis G. D., Shepard H. M. and Palladino M. A. jr. (1987): Inhibition of cytokine production by cyclosporin A and transforming growth factor beta. J. Exp. Med., **166**, 571–576.

Frei K., Eugster H. P., Bopst M., Constantinescu C. S., Lavi E. and Fontana A. (1997): Tumor necrosis factor alpha and lymphotoxin alpha are not required for induction of acute experimental autoimmune encephalomyelitis. J. Exp. Med., **185**, 2177–2182.

Gijbels K., Brocke S., Abrams J. S. and Steinman L. (1995): Administration of neutralizing antibodies to interleukin-6 (IL-6) reduces experimental autoimmune encephalomyelitis and is associated with elevated levels of IL-6 bioactivity in central nervous system and circulation. Mol. Med., **1**, 795–805.

Goverman J., Woods A., Larson L., Weiner L. P., Hood L. and Zaller D. M. (1993): Transgenic mice that express a myelin basic protein-specific T cell receptor develop spontaneous autoimmunity. Cell, **72**, 551–560.

Grewal I. S., Foellmer H. G., Grewal K. D., Xu J., Hardardottir F., Baron J. L., Janeway C. A. J. and Flavel R. A. (1996): Requirement for CD40 ligand in costimulation induction, T cell activation, and experimental allergic encephalomyelitis. Science, **273**, 1864–1867.

Groux H., O'Garra A., Bigler M., Rouleau M., Antonenko S., de Vries J. E. and Roncarlo M. G. (1997): A CD4+ T-cell subset inhibits antigen-specific T-cell responses and prevention colitis. Nature, **389**, 737–742.

Howard M., Farrar J., Hilfiker M., Johnson B., Takatsu K., Hamaoka T. and Paul W. E. (1982): Identification of a T cell-derived b cell growth factor distinct from interleukin 2. J. Exp. Med., **155**, 914–923.

Hsieh C. S., Heimberger A. B., Gold J. S., O'Garra A. and Murphy K. M. (1992): Differential regulation of T helper phenotype development by interleukins 4 and 10 in an alpha beta T-cell--receptor transgenic system. Proc. Natl. Acad. Sci. USA, **89**, 6065–6069.

Hsieh C. S., Macatonia S. E., Tripp C. S., Wolf S. F., O'Garra A. and Murphy K. M. (1993): Development of TH1 CD4+ T cells through IL-12 produced by *Listeria*-induced macrophages. Science, **260**, 547-549.

Inobe J. I., Chen Y. and Weiner H. L. (1996): *In vivo* administration of IL-4 induces TGF-beta--producing cells and protects animals from experimental autoimmune encephalomyelitis. Ann. NY Acad. Sci., **78**, 390–392.

Issazadeh S., Ljungdahl A., Hojeberg B., Mustafa M. and Olsson T. (1995): Cytokine production in the central nervous system of Lewis rats with experimental autoimmune encephalomyelitis: dynamics of mRNA expression for interleukin-10, interleukin-12, cytolysin, tumor necrosis factor alpha and tumor necrosis factor beta. J. Neuroimmunol., **61**, 205–212.

Issazedeh S., Lorentzen J. C., Mustafa M. I., Hojeberg B., Mussener A. and Olsson T. (1996): Cytokines in relapsing experimental autoimmune encephalomyelitis in DA rats: persistent mRNA expression of proinflammatory cytokines and absent expression of interleukin-10 and transforming growth factor-beta. J. Neuroimmunol., **69**, 103–115.

Jacobs C. A., Baker P. E., Roux E. R., Picha K. S., Toivola B., Waugh S. and Kennedy M. K. (1991): Experimental autoimmune encephalomyelitis is exacerbated by IL-1alpha and suppressed by soluble IL-1 receptor. J. Immunol., **146**, 2983–2989.

Johns L. D., Flanders K. C., Ranges G. E. and Sriram S. (1991): Successful treatment of experimental allergic encephalomyelitis with transforming growth factor-beta 1. J. Immunol., **147**, 1792–1796.

Kehrl J. H., Wakefield L. M., Roberts A. B., Jakowlew S., Alvarez-Mon M., Derynck R., Sporn M. B. and Fauci A. S. (1986): Production of transforming growth factor beta by human T lymphocytes and its potential role in the regulation of T cell growth. J. Exp. Med., **163**, 1037–1050.

Kennedy M. K., Torrance D. S., Picha K. S. and Mohler K. M. (1992): Analysis of cytokine mRNA expression in the central nervous system of mice with experimental autoimmune encephalomyelitis reveals that IL-10 mRNA expression correlates with recovery. J. Immunol., **149**, 2496–2505.

Khoury S. J., Hancock W. W. and Weiner H. L. (1992): Oral tolerance to myelin basic protein and natural recovery from experimental autoimmune encephalomyelitis are associated with downregulation of inflammatory cytokines and differential upregulation of transforming growth factor β, interleukin 4, and prostaglandin E expression in the brain. J. Exp. Med., **176**, 1355–1364.

Kivisakk P., Matusevicius D., He B., Soderstrom M., Fredrikson S. and Link H. (1998): IL-15 mRNA expression is up-regulated in blood and cerebrospinal fluid mononuclear cells in multiple sclerosis (MS). Clin. Exp. Immunol., **111**, 193–197.

Korner H., Lemckert F. A., Chaudhri G., Etteldorf S. and Sedgwick J. D. (1997a): Tumor necrosis factor blockade in actively induced experimental autoimmune encephalomyelitis prevents clinical disease despite activated T cell infiltration to the central nervous system. Eur. J. Immunol., **27**, 1973–1981.

Korner H., Riminton D. S., Strickland D. H., Lemckert F. A., Pollard J. D. and Sedgwick J. D. (1997b): Critical points of tumor necrosis factor action in central nervous system autoimmune inflammation defined by gene targeting. J. Exp. Med., **186**, 1585–1590.

Krakowski M. and Owens T. (1996): Interferon-gamma confers resistance to experimental allergic encephalomyelitis. Eur. J. Immunol., **26**, 1641–1646.

Kroemer G., Andreu J. L., Gonzalo J. A., Gutierrez-Ramos J. C. and Martinez A. C. (1991): Interleukin-2, autotolerance, and autoimmunity. Adv. Immunol., **50**, 147–235.

Kuchroo V. K., Prabhu Das M., Brown J. A., Ranger A. M., Zamvil S. S., Sobel R. A., Weiner H. L., Nabavi N. and Glimcher L. H. (1995): B7-1 and B7-2 costimulatory molecules activate differentially the Th1/Th2 developmental pathways: application to autoimmune disease therapy. Cell, **80**, 707–718.

Kuhn R., Rajewsky K. and Muller W. (1991): Generation and analysis of interleukin-4 deficient mice. Science, **254**, 707–710.

Kuruvilla A. P., Shah R., Hochwald G. M., Liggitt H. D., Palladino M. A. and Thorbecke G. J. (1991): Protective effect of transforming growth factor beta 1 on experimental autoimmune diseases in mice. Proc. Natl. Acad. Sci. USA, **88**, 2918–2921.

Lafaille J. J. (1998): The role of helper T cell subsets in autoimmune diseases. Cytokine Growth Factor Rev., **9**, 139–151.

Lafaille J. J., Nagashima K., Katsuki M. and Tonegawa S. (1994): High incidence of spontaneous autoimmune encephalomyelitis in immunodeficient anti-myelin basic protein T cell receptor transgenic mice. Cell, **78**, 399–408.

Lafaille J. J., van de Keere F., Hsu A. L., Baron J. L., Haas W., Raine C. S. and Tonegawa S. (1997): Myelin basic protein-specific T helper 2 (Th2) cells cause experimental autoimmune encephalomyelitis in immunodeficient hosts rather than protect them from the disease. J. Exp. Med., **186**, 307–312.

Leonard J. P., Waldburger K. E. and Goldman S. J. (1995): Prevention of experimental autoimmune encephalomyelitis by antibodies against interleukin 12. J. Exp. Med., **181**, 381–386.

Leonard J. P., Waldburger K. E. and Goldman S. J. (1996): Regulation of experimental autoimmune encephalomyelitis by interleukin-12. Ann. NY Acad. Sci., **795**, 216–226.

Liblau R., Steinman L. and Brocke S. (1997): Experimental autoimmune encephalomyelitis in IL-4-deficient mice. Int. Immunol., **9**, 799–803.

Liu J., Marino M. W., Wong G., Grail D., Dunn A., Bettadapura J., Slavin A. J., Old L. and Bernard C. C. (1998): TNF is a potent anti-inflammatory cytokine in autoimmune-mediated demyelination. Nat. Med., **4**, 78–83.

Mannie M. D., Dinarello C. A. and Paterson P. Y. (1987): Interleukin 1 and myelin basic protein synergistically augment adoptive transfer activity of lymphocytes mediating experimental autoimmune encephalomyelitis in Lewis rats. J. Immunol., **138**, 4229–4235.

Mathisen P. M., Yu M., Johnson J. M., Drazba J. A. and Tuohy V. K. (1997): Treatment of experimental autoimmune encephalomyelitis with genetically modified memory T cells. J. Exp. Med., **186**, 159–164.

Mendel I., Katz A., Kozak N., Ben-Nun A. and Revel M. (1998): Interleukin-6 functions in autoimmune encephalomyelitis: a study in gene-targeted mice. Eur. J. Immunol., **28**, 1727–1737.

Merrill J. E., Kono D. H., Clayton J., Ando D. G., Hinton D. R. and Hofman F. M. (1992): Inflammatory leukocytes and cytokines in the peptide-induced disease of experimental allergic encephalomyelitis in SJL and B10. PL mice [published erratum appears in Proc. Natl. Acad. Sci. USA 1992 Nov 1; 89(21): 10562]. Proc. Natl. Acad. Sci. USA, **89**, 574–578.

Micallef M. J., Ohtsuki T., Kohno K., Tanabe F., Ushio S., Namba M., Tanimoto, Torigoe K., Fujii M., Ikeda M., Fukuda S. and Kurimoto M. (1996): Interferon-gamma-inducing factor enhances T helper 1 cytokine production by stimulated human T cells: synergism with interleukin-12 for interferon-gamma production. Eur. J. Immunol., **26**, 1647–1651.

Miller A., Lider O., Roberts A. B., Sporn M. B. and Weiner H. L. (1992): Suppressor T cells generated by oral tolerization to myelin basic protein suppress both *in vitro* and *in vivo* immune responses by the release of transforming growth factor β after antigen-specific triggering. Proc. Natl. Acad. Sci. USA, **89**, 421–425.

Mosmann T. R. and Sad S. (1996): The expanding universe of T-cell subsets: Th1, Th2 and more. Immunol. Today, **17**, 138–146.

Nagelkerken L., Blauw B. and Tielemans M. (1997): IL-4 abrogates the inhibitory effect of IL-10 on the development of experimental allergic encephalomyelitis in SJL mice [published erratum appears in Int. Immunol. 1997 Nov; 9(11): 1773]. Int. Immunol., **9**, 1243–1251.

Nicholson L. B., Carrizosa A. M. and Kuchroo V. K. (1998): Pathogenic versus protective repertoires in autoimmune disease: Tuning the balance. Immunologist, **6**, 151–157.

Nicholson L. B. and Kuchroo V. K. (1996): Manipulation of the Th1/Th2 balance in autoimmune disease. Curr. Opin. Immunol., **8**, 837–842.

Nicholson L. B., Murtaza A., Hafler B. P., Sette A. and Kuchroo V. K. (1997a): A T cell receptor antagonist peptide prevents autoimmune encephalomyelitis induced with multiple myelin antigens: Evidence for bystander suppression. Proc. Natl. Acad. Sci. USA, **94**, 9279–9284.

Nicholson L. B., Windhagen A., Prabhu Das M., Hafler D. A. and Kuchroo V. K. (1997b): The role of immune deviation in regulation of experimental autoimmune encephalomyelitis and multiple sclerosis. In Adorini L. (ed.): Immunointervention in autoimmunity by Th1/Th2 regulation. Landes Bioscience, Austin, Texas, 105–127.

Okuda Y., Nakatsuji Y., Fujimura H., Esumi H., Ogura T., Yanagihara T. and Sakoda S. (1995): Expression of the inducible isoform of nitric oxide synthase in the central nervous system of mice correlates with the severity of actively induced experimental allergic encephalomyelitis. J. Neuroimmunol., **62**, 103–112.

Okuda Y., Sakoda S., Bernard C. C., Fujimura H., Saeki Y., Kishimoto T. and Yanagihara T. (1998): IL-6-deficient mice are resistant to the induction of experimental autoimmune encephalomyelitis provoked by myelin oligodendrocyte glycoprotein. Int. Immunol., **10**, 703–708.

Panitch H. S. and Bever C. T. Jr. (1993): Clinical trials of interferons in multiple sclerosis. What have we learned? J. Neuroimmunol., **46**, 155–164.

Pohl-Koppe A., Balashov K. E., Steere A. C., Logigian E. L. and Hafler D. A. (1998): Identification of a T cell subset capable of both IFN-gamma and IL-10 secretion in patients with chronic *Borrelia burgdorferi* infection. J. Immunol., **160**, 1804–1810.

Powell H. C., Garrett R. S., Brett F. M., Chiang C. S., Chen E., Masliah E. and Campbell I. L. (1999): Response of glia, mast cells and the blood brain barrier, in transgenic mice expressing interleukin-3 in astrocytes, an experimental model for CNS demyelination. Brain Pathol., **9**, 219–235.

Racke M. K., Bonomo A., Scott D. E., Cannella B., Levine A., Raine C. S., Shevach E. M. and Rocken M. (1994): Cytokine-induced immune deviation as a therapy for inflammatory autoimmune disease. J. Exp. Med., **180**, 1961–1966.

Racke M. K., Cannella B., Albert P., Sporn M., Raine C. S. and McFarlin D. E. (1992): Evidence of endogenous regulatory function of transforming growth factor-beta 1 in experimental allergic encephalomyelitis. Int. Immunol., **4**, 615–620.

Racke M. K., Dhib-Jalbut S., Cannella B., Albert P. S., Raine C. S. and McFarlin D. E. (1991): Prevention and treatment of chronic relapsing experimental allergic encephalomyelitis by transforming growth factor-beta 1. J. Immunol., **146**, 3012–3017.

Reiner S. L., Wang Z., Hatam F., Scott P. and Locksley R. M. (1993): Th1 and Th2 cell antigen receptors in experimental leishmaniasis. Science, **259**, 1457–1460.

Robinson D., Shibuya K., Mui A., Zonin F., Murphy E., Sana T., Hartley S. B., Menon S., Kastelein R., Bazan F. and O'Garra A. (1997): IGIF does not drive Th1 development but synergizes with IL-12 for interferon-gamma production and activates IRAK and NFkappaB. Immunity, **7**, 571–581.

Rodriguez M., Pavelko K. D., McKinney C. W. and Leibowitz J. L. (1994): Recombinant human IL-6 suppressed demyelination in a viral model of multiple sclerosis. J. Immunol., **153**, 3811–3821.

Romagnani S. (1994): Lymphokine production by human T cells in disease states. Annu. Rev. Immunol., **12**, 227–257.

Romani L., Mencacci A., Grohmann U., Mocci S., Mosci P., Puccetti P. and Bistoni F. (1992): Neutralizing antibody to interleukin 4 induces systemic protection and T helper type 1-associated immunity in murine candidiasis. J. Exp. Med., **176**, 19–25.

Rott O., Fleischer B. and Cash E. (1994): Interleukin-10 prevents experimental allergic encephalomyelitis in rats. Eur. J. Immunol., **24**, 1434–1440.

Ruckert R., Herz U., Paus R., Ungureanu D., Pohl T., Renz H. and Bulfone-Paus S. (1998): IL-15-IgG2b fusion protein accelerates and enhances a Th2 but not a Th1 immune response *in vivo*, while IL-2-IgG2b fusion protein inhibits both. Eur. J. Immunol., **28**, 3312–3320.

Ruddle N. H., Bergman C. M., McGrath K. M., Lingenheld E. G., Grunnet M. L., Padula S. J. and Clark R. B. (1990): An antibody to lymphotoxin and tumor necrosis factor prevents transfer of experimental allergic encephalomyelitis. J. Exp. Med., **172**, 1193–1200.

Sadlack B., Lohler J., Schorle H., Klebb G., Haber H., Sickel E., Noelle R. J. and Horak I. (1995): Generalized autoimmune disease in interleukin-2-deficient mice is triggered by an uncontrolled activation and proliveration of CD4+ T cells. Eur. J. Immunol., **25**, 3053–3059.

Sadlack B., Merz H., Schorle H., Schimpl A., Feller A. C. and Horak I. (1993): Ulcerative colitis-like disease in mice with a disrupted interleukin-2 gene. Cell, **75**, 253–261.

Samoilova E. B., Horton J. L. and Chen Y. (1998a): Acceleration of experimental autoimmune encephalomyelitis in interleukin-10-deficient mice: roles of interleukin-10 in disease progression and recovery. Cell. Immunol., **188**, 118–124.

Samoilova E. B., Horton J. L., Hillard B., Liu T. S. and Chen Y. (1998b): IL-6-deficient mice are resistant to experimental autoimmune encephalomyelitis: roles of IL-6 in the activation and differentiation of autoreactive T cells. J. Immunol., **161**, 6480–6486.

Santambrogio L., Hochwald G. M., Saxena B., Leu C. H., Martz J. E., Carlino J. A., Ruddle N. H., Palladino M. A., Gold L. I. and Thorbecke G. J. (1993): Studies on the mechanisms by which transforming growth factor-beta (TGF-beta) protects against allergic encephalomyelitis. Antagonism between TGF-beta and tumor necrosis factor. J. Immunol., **151**, 1116–1127.

Schluesener H. J. (1990): Transforming growth factors type beta 1 and beta 2 suppress rat astrocyte autoantigen presentation and antagonize hyperinduction of class II major histocompatibility complex antigen expression by interferon-gamma and tumor necrosis factor-alpha. J. Neuroimmunol., **27**, 41–47.

Seder R. A., Gazzinelli R., Sher A. and Paul W. E. (1993): Interleukin 12 acts directly on CD4+ T cells to enhance priming for interferon gamma production and diminishes interleukin 4 inhibition of such priming. Proc. Natl. Acad. Sci. USA, **90**, 10188–10192.

Seder R. A., Paul W. E., Davis M. M. and Fazekas de St. Groth B. (1992): The presence of interleukin 4 during *in vitro* priming determines the lymphokine-producing potential of CD4+ T cell from receptor transgenic mice. J. Exp. Med., **176**, 1091–1098.

Segal B. M., Dwyer B. K. and Shevach E. M. (1998): An interleukin (IL)-10/IL-12 immunoregulatory circuit controls susceptibility to autoimmune disease. J. Exp. Med., **187**, 537–546.

Selmaj K., Raine C. S. and Cross A. H. (1991): Anti-tumor necrosis factor therapy abrogates autoimmune demyelination. Ann. Neurol., **30**, 694–700.

Shaw M. K., Lorens J. B., Dhawan A., Dal Canto R., Tse H. Y., Tran A. B., Bonpane C., Eswaran S. L., Brocke S., Sarvetnick N., Steinmar L., Nolan G. P. and Fathman C. G. (1997): Local delivery of interleukin 4 by retrovirus-transduced T lymphocytes ameliorates experimental autoimmune encephalomyelitis. J. Exp. Med., **185**, 1711–1714.

Smith K. A. (1988): Interleukin-2: inception, impact, and implications. Science, **240**, 1169–1176.

Sobel R. A., Green J. A. and Kuchroo V. K. (1994): Autoimmune responses to myelin proteolipid protein. Neurochem. Res., **19**, 915–921.

Steinman L. (1997): Some misconceptions about understanding autoimmunity through experiments with knockouts. J. Exp. Med., **185**, 2039–2041.

Suen W. E., Bergman C. M., Hjelmstrom P. and Ruddle N. H. (1997): A critical role for lymphotoxin in experimental allergic encephalomyelitis. J. Exp. Med., **186**, 1233–1240.

Swain S. L., Weinberg A. D., English M. and Huston G. (1990): IL-4 directs the development of Th2-like helper effectors. J. Immunol., **145**, 3796–3806.

Taga T. and Kishimoto T. (1997): Gp130 and the interleukin-6 family of cytokines. Annu. Rev. Immunol., **15**, 797–819.

Tanuma N., Kojima T., Shin T., Aikawa Y., Kohji T., Ishihara Y. and Matsumoto Y. (1997): Competitive PCR quantification of pro- and anti-inflammatory cytokine mRNA in the central nervous system during autoimmune encephalomyelitis. J. Neuroimmunol., **73**, 197–206.

The Lenercept Multiple Sclerosis Study Group (1999): TNF neutralization in MS: Results of a randomized, placebo-controlled multicenter study. Neurology, **53**, 457–465.

Trinchieri G. and Scott P. (1995): Interleukin-12: a proinflammatory cytokine with immunoregulatory functions. Res. Immunol., **146**, 423–431.

Tsunawaki S., Sporn M., Ding A. and Nathan C. (1988): Deactivation of macrophages by transforming growth factor-beta. Nature, **334**, 260–262.

Van Oosten B. W., Barkhof F., Truyen L., Boringa J. B., Bertelsmann F. W., von Blomberg B. M., Woody J. N., Hartung H. P. and Polman C. H. (1996): Increased MRI activity and immune activation in two multiple sclerosis patients treated with the monoclonal anti-tumor necrosis factor antibody cA2. Neurology, **47**, 1531–1534.

Van Parijs L. and Abbas A. (1998): Homeostatis and self-tolerance in the immune system-turning lymphocytes off. Science, **280**, 243–248.

Waksman B. H. (1995): Multiple sclerosis. More genes versus environment. Nature, **377**, 105–106.

Waldmann T. A. and Tagaya Y. (1999): The multifaceted regulation of interleukin-15 expression and the role of this cytokine in NK cell differentiation and host response to intracellular pathogens. Annu. Rev. Immunol., **17**, 19–49.

Waldner H.-P., Whitters M. J., Sobel R. A., Collins M. and Kuchroo V. K. (2000): Fulminant spontaneous autoimmunity of the central nervous system in myelin proteolipid protein specific T cell receptor transgenic mice. Proc. Natl. Acad. Sci. USA, **97**, 3412–3417.

Wekerle H. (1993): Experimental autoimmune encephalomyelitis as a model of immune-mediated CNS disease. Curr. Opin. Neurobiol., **3**, 779–784.

Wildbaum G., Youssef S., Grabie N. and Karin N. (1998): Neutralizing antibodies to IFN-gamma-inducing factor prevent experimental autoimmune encephalomyelitis. J. Immunol., **161**, 6368–6374.

Willenborg D. O., Fordham S. A., Cowden W. B. and Ramshaw I. A. (1995): Cytokines and murine autoimmune encephalomyelitis: inhibition or enhancement of disease with antibodies to select cytokines, or by delivery of exogenous cytokines using a recombinant vaccinia virus system. Scand. J. Immunol., **41**, 31–41.

Willenborg D. O., Fordham S. A., O'Brien N. C., Cowden W. B. and Ramshaw I. A. (1998): Tumor necrosis factor-alpha and lymphotoxin alpha in the pathology of experimental autoimmune encephalomyelitis: is either one responsible or is there another ligand mediating disease. Res. Immunol., **149**, 804–810.

Zamvil S. S. and Steinman L. (1990): The T lymphocyte in experimental allergic encephalomyelitis. Annu. Rev. Immunol., **8**, 579–621.

Zhang B., Yamamura T., Kondo T., Fujiwara M. and Tabira T. (1997): Regulation of experimental autoimmune encephalomyelitis by natural killer (NK) cells. J. Exp. Med., **186**, 1677–1687.

INVOLVEMENT OF APOPTOTIC PROTEASE CASCADE FOR TISSUE DESTRUCTION IN SJÖGREN'S SYNDROME

YOSHIO HAYASHI

Department of Pathology, Tokushima University School of Dentistry, 3 Kuramotocho, Tokushima 770, Japan

Abstract Sjögren syndrome (SS) is an autoimmune disease characterized by diffuse lymphoid cell infiltrates in the salivary and lacrimal glands, resulting in symptoms of dry mouth and eyes due to insufficient secretion. Although it has been assumed that a combination of immunologic, genetic and environmental factors may play a key role in the development of autoimmune lesions in the salivary and lacrimal glands, little is known about the disease pathogenesis of SS in humans. We have identified the 120 kDa α-fodrin as an important autoantigen in the development of SS in both an animal model and SS patients, but the mechanism of α-fodrin cleavage leading to tissue destruction in SS remains unclear. Tissue-infiltrating $CD4^+$ T cells purified from the salivary glands of a mouse model for SS bear a large proportion of Fas ligand and the salivary gland duct cells possess apoptotic receptor Fas. Anti-Fas antibody-induced apoptotic salivary gland cells result in specific α-fodrin cleavage to the 120 kDa fragment *in vitro*. Preincubation with a combination of calpain and caspase inhibitor peptides could be responsible for inhibition of the 120 kDa α-fodrin cleavage. Thus, an increase in apoptotic protease activities including calpain and caspases may be involved in the progression of α-fodrin proteolysis and tissue destruction in the development of SS.

Key words: Sjögren's syndrome; autoantigen; protease; apoptosis.

1. INTRODUCTION

Sjögren's syndrome (SS) is a chronic autoimmune disorder affecting the salivary and lacrimal glands and leads to the clinical symptoms of dryness of the mouth and eyes (sicca syndrome) (Bloch et al., 1965). The histopathological changes in the minor salivary gland biopsy are characterized by focal and/or diffuse lymphoid cell infiltrates and parenchymal destruction. The

A. Górski et al. (eds.), Autoimmunity, 129–137.

majority of lymphoid cells in the salivary biopsy are $CD4^+$ T cells, with a small proportion of $CD8^+$ T cells (Fox and Saito, 1995). These T cells express the αb antigen receptor and cell surface antigens associated with mature memory T cells. Since a preferential use of specific variable region segments of the antigen receptor β chain by salivary gland T cells was evident (Sumida et al., 1992), it has been assumed that an unknown organ-specific autoantigen targeted by autoreactive T cells may be present in the salivary glands.

We have established an animal model for primary SS in NFS/*sld* mutant mice thymectomized 3 day after birth (3d-Tx) (Haneji et al., 1994; Hayashi et al., 1988). When the repertoire of T cell receptor (TCR) Vβ genes transcribed and expressed within the inflammatory infiltrates was analyzed in the animal model, a preferential utilization of TCR Vβ gene was detected in these lesions from the onset of disease (Haneji et al., 1994). We have recently identified a 120 kDa organ-specific autoantigen from the salivary gland tissues of this animal model. The sequence of the first 20 NH_2-terminal residues was found to be identical to that of cytoskeletal protein human α-fodrin (Haneji et al., 1997). Furthermore, sera from patients with SS reacted positively with purified 120 kDa antigen, and proliferative response of peripheral blood lymphocytes (PBMC) from SS patients to the purified autoantigen was detected, but not from systematic lupus erythematosis (SLE) or rheumatoid arthitris (RA) patients and healthy controls. These results indicate that the anti-120 kDa α-fodrin immune response plays an essential role in the development of primary SS.

Autoimmune diseases are characterized by tissue destruction and functional decline due to autoreactive T cells that escape self-tolerance (Feldmann et al., 1996; Gianani and Satventnick, 1989). Although the specificity of the cytotoxic T lymphocyte (CTL) function has been an important issue of organ--specific autoimmune response, the mechanisms responsible for tissue destruction in SS remain to be elucidated (Chan et al., 1991; Kruize et al., 1995). It is now clear that the interaction of Fas with Fas ligand (FasL) regulates a large number of the pathophysiological proceses of apoptosis (Brunner et al., 1995; Ju et al., 1995). We speculate that an increase in the enzymatic activity of apoptotic proteases is involved in the progression of α-fodrin proteolysis during the development of SS.

2. INVOLVEMENT OF FAS AND FASL IN TISSUE DESTRUCTION

To determine the possible involvement of Fas and FasL in the tissue destruction of SS, we first analyzed Fas expression in the salivary gland specimens of the 3d-Tx NFS/*sld* mouse model (Haneji et al., 1994) and in the mouse salivary gland cells (MSG) isolated from non-thymectomized (non-Tx) NFS/*sld* mice. Immunohistochemistry revealed that epithelial duct cells express a large amount of Fas on their cell surface in 3d-Tx NFS/*sld* mice, also detected by *in situ* TUNEL assay. However, we found that epithelial duct cells in non-Tx NFS/*sld* and normal salivary glands are constitutively positive for Fas, but not for TUNEL staining, suggesting that Fas expression does not correlate with its apoptotic function in normal salivary gland cells. Isolated MSG cells express Fas with high proportion (>66%) on FACS staining (Fig. 1). We found that the tissue-infiltrating $CD4^+$ T cells purified from the salivary gland tissues of 3d-Tx NFS/*sld* mice bear a large proportion of FasL (>73%) (Fig. 1). Immunohistochemical analysis revealed that FasL expression was completely absent on the salivary gland epithelial cells in any strain of mouse. RT-PCR analysis demonstrated that Fas mRNA was present in both salivary glands, and a high level of FasL mRNA was detected in the salivary glands of 3d-Tx NFS/*sld* mice, but not in non-Tx and normal mice. Protein immunoblot analysis confirmed the expression of FasL in salivary glands of 3d-Tx NFS/*sld* mice.

We next investigated whether activated $CD4^+$ T cells are responsible for tissue destruction as judged by *in vitro* ^{51}Cr release cytotoxic assay against MSG cells. MSG cells (2×10^6) in 7.5 ml of MEM were labeled overnight at 37°C in 5% CO_2 with 300 μCi of sodium [^{51}Cr]-chromate. $CD4^+$ and $CD8^+$ T cells purified from splenocytes using magnetic beads were incubated with ConA and recombinant human IL-2. The splenic $CD4^+$ T cells activated with ConA and IL-2 showed significant ^{51}Cr release against MSG cells (Fig. 2). These cytotoxic activities were almost entirely inhibited by incubation with anti-murine neutralizing FasL antibody, indicating that the cytotoxicity by

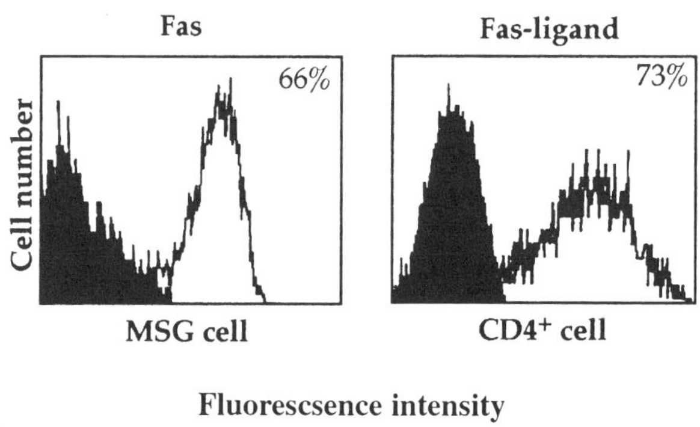

Figure 1. Flow cytometric analysis of Fas expression on mouse salivary gland (MSG) cells and FasL expression on the tissue-infiltrating lymphocytes purified from affected salivary glands of animal model for Sjögren's syndrome gated on CD4

activated CD4+ T cells towards salivary gland epithelial cells was Fas--based.

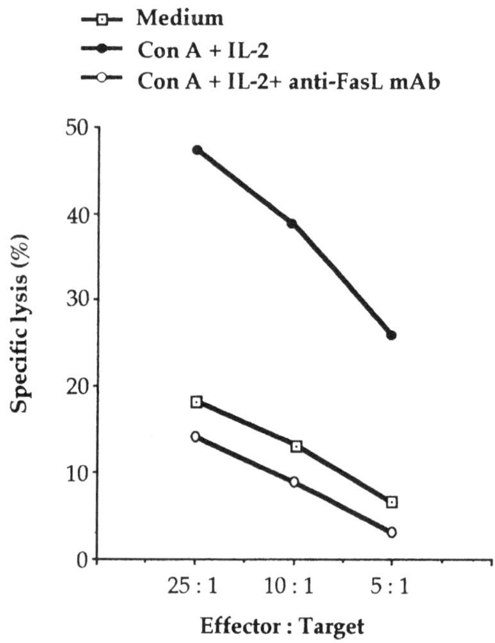

Figure 2. Cytotoxic activity of activated CD4+ T cells from spleen towards Fas-sensitive MSG cells. Splenic CD4+ T cells activated with ConA and IL-2 identified significant ^{51}Cr release against MSG cells. This activity was almost entirely inhibited by anti-murine neutralizing FasL antibody

3. PARTICIPATION OF CALPAIN AND CASPASES IN α-FODRIN CLEAVAGE

To confirm the organ-specificity of a cleavage product of α-fodrin, we investigated various strains of mice with salivary gland destruction, such as MRL/*lpr* non-obese diabetic (NOD) mice, in addition to 3d-TX NFS/*sld* mice. Protein immunoblot analysis demonstrated that the 120 kDa α-fodrin was detected in these affected glands, but not in normal mice. We examined the *in vitro* cleavage of α-fodrin using 240 kDa α-fodrin in MSG cells. Anti--Fas antibody (Ab)-induced apoptosis was confirmed by FACS analysis using the *in situ* TUNEL procedure and by DNA laddering and formation. We could detect the 120 kDa α-fodrin in apoptotic MSG cells on immunoblotting. Similar evidence was obtained with a human salivary gland (HSG) epithelial cell line (Shirasuna et al., 1981). Apoptotic HSG cells induced by treatment with anti-Fas Ab was confirmed. Immunoblot analysis demonstrated that the 240 kDa α-fodrin on apoptotic HSG cells was cleaved to smaller fragments, including 150 kDa and 120 kDa (Fig. 3).

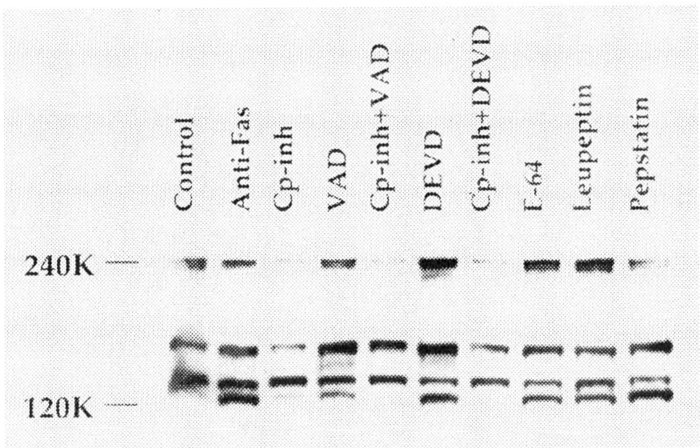

Figure 3. Protein immunoblot analysis of 120 kDa α-fodrin in apoptotic human salivary gland (HSG) cells treated with anti-Fas mAb. 120 kDa α-fodrin was detected in apoptotic HSG cells

We next investigated whether cysteine proteases are involved in α-fodrin cleavage on apoptotic HSG cells. Anti-Fas Ab treated HSG cells were positive for mAb to μ-calpain, and to ICE (p20) and CPP32 in association with apoptosis. The ICE- and CPP32-like activities in anti-Fas Ab treated HSG cell extracts were then determined using fluorescent substrates (Enari et al., 1996). The specific inhibitor for ICE (Ac-YVAD-cmk) or CPP32 (Z-DEVD--fmk) was added to the reaction mixture at a concentration of 1 μM. Specific ICE- and CPP32-like activities were determined by subtracting the values obtained in the presence of inhibitors. These results suggest that protease families including calpain and caspases participate in the progression of α-fodrin cleavage of apoptotic HSG cells.

4. PREVENTIVE EFFECT OF CASPASE INHIBITOR *IN VIVO*

To address this hypothesis, we examined whether α-fodrin cleavage to the 120 kDa fragment on apoptotic HSG cells could be blocked by preincubation with specific protease inhibitors. In apoptotic HSG cells, calpain inhibitor peptide and caspase inhibitor (Z-VAD-fmk) had partially blocked 120 kDa α-fodrin formation. Moreover, a combination of calpain inhibitor peptide and caspase inhibitors (Z-VAD-fmk and Z-DEVD-fmk) almost entirely inhibited the formation of 120 kDa α-fodrin. Protease inhibitor cocktails, other cysteine protease inhibitors (E-64) and serine protease inhibitor (Leupeptin) had no effect on 120 kDa α-fodrin cleavage in apoptotic HSG cells. The specificity of a combination of calpain and caspase inhibitors towards the decrease in 120 kDa α-fodrin in the HSG cells will be further quantified in detail.

By immunohistochemistry using polyclonal Ab against synthetic 120 kDa α-fodrin, a cleavage product of α-fodrin was present exclusively in epithelial duct cells of the labial salivary gland biopsies from SS patients, but not in control individuals. Protein immunoblot analysis confirmed the same results. This indicates that a cleavage product of 120 kDa α-fodrin is present in the diseased glands with human SS, but not in control glands. We next investigated whether the intravenous injection of caspase inhibitor, Z-VAD-fmk, protects animals against the development of autoimmune lesions. The treatment with intravenous injection of Z-VAD-fmk prevented the development of autoimmune conditions including lymphocytic infiltration and autoantibody production to the whole 120 kDa molecule.

5. PERSPECTIVE

Although cleavage of certain autoantigens during apoptosis may reveal immunocryptic epitopes that could potentially induce autoimmune responses in systemic autoimmune diseases (Casiano, 1996; Utz et al., 1997), no evidence whether *in vivo* cleavage of autoantigen occurs in organ-specific autoimmune diseases has yet been described. The roles of the Fas/FasL system in the pathogenesis of autoimmune diseases have already been proposed (Bieganowska et al., 1997; Nagata and Goldstein, 1995; Nishio et al., 1996; Rieux-Laucat, 1995; Saito et al., 1999; Thompson, 1995). It has been recently reported that both Fas and FasL are present in thyrocytes and their concomitant expression on thyrocytes, independent of infiltrating T cells, is responsible for thyrocyte destruction in Hashimoto's thyroiditis (Giordano et al., 1997). In contrast, expression of Fas by pancreatic β cells has been shown to have a major influence on the susceptibility of tissue destruction in NOD mice to diabetes (Chervonsky et al., 1997). In this study, we provide evidence suggesting that Fas/FasL-mediated apoptosis may be involved in the initial cascade of the *in vivo* cleavage of autoantigen and that $CD4^+$ cytotoxic T cells may participate in the tissue destruction of SS salivary glands.

When human T cell leukemia CEM cells were induced to undergo apoptosis, the 240 kDa α-fodrin was cleaved to a single detectable fragment of 120 kDa (Patel et al., 1996). It was plausible that the 120 kD fragment is a break-down product of the 150 kDa α-fodrin cleavage (Martin et al., 1995). The analysis of proteolytic events associated with apoptosis is to define the mechanisms leading to protease activation and to identify key substrates whose cleavage might be linked to the profound changes in cellular architecture. There is increasing evidence that calpain is overactivated in autoimmune conditions and subsequent tissue destruction (Menad and El-Amine, 1996; Mimori et al., 1995). Moreover, the cascade of caspases is a critical component of the cell death pathway (Holtzman and Deshmukh, 1997; Huang et al., 1997; Kothakota et al., 1997; Rudel and Bokoch, 1997) and a few proteins have been found to be cleaved during apoptosis. These include poly (ADP-ribose) polymerase (PARP), a small U1 nuclear ribonucleoprotein (RNP), and α-fodrin, which were subsequently identified as substrates for caspases (Casiano et al., 1996). We provided evidence that α-fodrin is not only cleaved by calpain, but also by one or more members of the caspases during Fas/FasL mediated-apoptosis in SS salivary glands. Fodrin cleavage by calpain and caspases can potentially lead to cytoskeltal derangement. Above all, it is of great interest to point out that α-fodrin binds to ankylin, which contains a cell death domain (Feinstein et al., 1995).

In conclusion, these results are strongly suggestive of a role for calpain- and caspase-mediated cleavage of α-fodrin in the functional activation of autoreactive T cells in SS, and could be consistent with a role for Fas/FasL--mediated apoptosis in the development of autoimmune tissue destruction. Moreover, *in vivo* preventive effects against autoimmune lesions treated with protease inhibitors have important implications for testing useful therapies.

REFERENCES

Bieganowska K. D., Ausubel L. J., Modabber Y., Slovik E., Messersmith W. and Hafler D. A. (1997): Direct *ex vivo* analysis of activated, Fas-sensitive autoreactive T cells in human autoimmune disease. J. Exp. Med., **185**, 1585–1594.

Bloch K. J., Buchanan W. W., Wohl M. J. and Bunim J. (1965): Sjögen's syndrome. A clinical, pathological and serological study of sixty-two cases. Medicine, **44**, 187–231.

Brunner T., Mogll R. J., La Face D., Yoo N. J., Mahboubl A., Echeverri F., Martin S. J., Force W. R., Lynch D. H., Ware C. F. and Green D. R. (1995): Cell-autonomous Fas (CD95)/Fas-ligand interaction mediates activation-induced apoptosis in T cell hybridomas. Nature, **373**, 441–444.

Casiano C. A. (1996): Selective cleavage of nuclear autoantigens during CD95 (Fas/APO-1)--mediated T cell apoptosis. J. Exp. Med., **184**, 765–770.

Casiano C. A., Martin S. J., Green D. R. and Tan E. T. (1996): Selective cleavage of nuclear autoantigens during CD95 (Fas/APO-1)-mediated T cell apoptosis. J. Exp. Med., **184**, 765–770.

Chan E. K., Hamel J. C., Buyon J. P. and Tan E. T. (1991): Molecular definition and sequence motifs of the 52-kD component of human SS-A/Ro autoantigen. J. Clin. Invest., **87**, 68–76.

Chervonsky A. V., Wang Y., Wong F. S., Visintin I., Flavell R. A., Janeway C. A. Jr. and Matis L. A. (1997): The role of Fas in autoimmune diabetes. Cell, **89**, 17–24.

Enari M., Talanian R. V., Wong W. W. and Nagata S. (1996): Sequential activation of ICE-loke and CPP32-like proteases during Fas-mediated apoptosis. Nature, **380**, 723–726.

Feinstein E., Kimchi A., Wallach D., Boldin M. and Varfolomeev E. (1995): The death domain: a module shared by proteins with diverse cellular function. Trends Biochem. Sci., **20**, 342–344.

Feldmann M., Bennan F. M. and Maini R. N. (1996): Rheumatoid arthritis. Cell, **85**, 307–310.

Fox R. I. and Saito I. (1995): Sjögren's syndrome. In Robert R. (ed.): Clinical immunology-principles and practice. Chapter 75. Mosby, 1145–1153.

Gianani R. and Satventnick N. (1989): Virus, cytokine, antigens, and autoimmunity. Proc. Natl. Acad. Sci. USA, **93**, 2252–2259.

Giordano C., Stassi G., De Maria R., Todaro M., Richiusa P., Papoff G., Ruberti G., Bagnasco M., Testi R. and Galluzzo A. (1997): Potential involvement of Fas and its ligand in the pathogenesis of Hashimoto's thyroiditis. Science, **275**, 960–963.

Haneji N., Hamono H., Yanagi K. and Hayashi Y. (1994): A new animal model for primary Sjögren's syndrome in NFS/*sld* mutant mice. J. Immunol., **153**, 2769–2777.

Haneji N., Nakamura T., Takio K., Yanagi K., Higashiyama H., Saito I., Noji S., Sugino H. and Hayashi Y. (1997): Identification of α-fodrin as a candidate autoantigen in primary Sjögren's syndrome. Science, **276**, 604–607.

Hayashi Y., Kojima A., Hata M. and Hirokawa K. (1988): A new mutationinvolving the sublingual gland in NFS/N mice. Am. J. Pathol., **132**, 187–191.

Holtzman D. M. and Deshmukh M. (1997): Caspases: A treatment target for neurodegenerative disease? Nat. Med., **3**, 954–955.

Huang S., Jiang Y., Li Z., Nishida E., Mathias P., Lin S., Ulevitch R. J., Nemerow G. R. and Han J. (1997): Apoptosis signaling pathway in T cells is composed of ICE/Ced-3 familiy proteases and MAP kinase 6b. Immunity, **6**, 739–749.

Ju S.-T., Panka D. J., Cui H., Ettinger R., El-Khatib M., Sherr D. H., Stanger B. Z. and Marshak-Rothstein A. (1995): Fas(CD95)/FasL interactions required for programmed cell death after T-cell activation. Nature, **373**, 444–448.

Kothakota S., Azuma T., Reinhard C., Klippel A., Tang J., Chu K., McGarry T. J., Kirschner M. W., Koths K., Kwiatkowski D. J. and Williams L. T. (1997): Caspase-3-generated fragment of Gelsolin: Effector of morphological change in apoptosis. Science, **278**, 294–298.

Kruize A. A., Smeenk R. J. T. and Kater L. (1995): Diagnostic criteria and immunopathogenesis of Sjögren's syndrome: implications for therapy. Immunol. Today, **16**, 557–559.

Martin S. D., O'Brien G. A., Nishioka W. K., McGahon A. J., Mahboubi A., Saido T. C. and

Green D. R. (1995): Proteolysis of fodrin (non-erythroid spectrin) during apoptosis. J. Biol. Chem., **270**, 6425–6428.

Menad H.-A. and El-Amine M. (1996): The calpain-calpastatin system in rheumatoid arthritis. Immunol. Today, **17**, 545–547.

Mimori T., Suganuma K., Tanami Y., Nojima T., Matsumura M., Fujii T., Yoshizawa T., Suzuki K. and Akizuki M. (1995): Autoantibodies to calpastatin (an endogenous inhibitor for calcium-dependent neutral protease, calpain) in systemic rheumatic diseases. Proc. Natl. Acad. Sci. USA, **92**, 7267–7271.

Nagata S. and Goldstein P. (1995): The Fas death factor. Science, **267**, 1449–1456.

Nishio A., Katakai T., Oshima C., Kasakura S., Sakai M., Yonehara S., Suda T., Nagata S. and Masuda T. (1996): A possible involvement of Fas-Fas ligand signaling in the pathogenesis of murine autoimmune gastritis. Gastroenterology, **111**, 956–967.

Patel T., Gores G. J. and Kaufmann S. H. (1996): The role of proteases during apoptosis. FASEB J., **10**, 587–597.

Rieux-Laucat F. (1995): Mutation in Fas associated with human lymphoproliferative syndrome and autoimmunity. Science, **268**, 1347–1349.

Rudel T. and Bokoch G. M. (1997): Membrane and morphological changes in apoptotic cells regulated by caspase-mediated activation of PAK2. Science, **276**, 1571–1574.

Saito I., Haruta K., Shimuta M., Inoue H., Sakurai H., Yamada K., Ishimaru N., Higashiyama H., Sumida T., Ishida H., Suda T., Noda T., Hayashi Y. and Tshubota K. (1999): Fas ligand-mediated excrinopathy resembling Sjögren's syndrome in mice transgenic for IL-10. J. Immunol., **162**, 2488–2494.

Shirasuna K., Sato M. and Miyazaki T. (1981): A neoplastic epithelial duct cell line established from an irradiated human salivary gland. Cancer, **48**, 745–752.

Sumida T., Yonaha F., Maeda T., Tanabe E., Koike T., Tomioka H. and Yoshida S. (1992): T cell receptor repertoire of infiltrating T cells in lips of Sjögren's syndrome patients. J. Clin. Invest., **89**, 681–685.

Thompson C. B. (1995): Apoptosis in the pathogenesis and treatment of disease. Science, **267**, 1456–1462.

Utz P. J., Hottelet M., Schur P. H. and Anderson P. (1997): Proteins phospholylated during stress-induced apoptosis are common targets for autoantibody production in patients with systemic lupus erythematosus. J. Exp. Med., **185**, 843–854.

IS LACK OF PERIPHERAL TOLERANCE INDUCTION A CAUSE FOR DIABETES IN THE NON-OBESE DIABETIC MOUSE?

TORBEN LUND[1] and JESSICA STRID[2]

[1] *Department of Immunology and Molecular Pathology, Windeyer Institute for Medical Sciences*
[2] *Immunobiology Unit, Institute of Child Health, University College London, London, UK*

Abstract The non-obese diabetic (NOD) mouse is a spontaneous animal model for type 1 diabetes characterized by a selective destruction of the insulin producing β cells in the pancreas. As in humans, the disease is controlled by several susceptibility genes, some of which map to the major histocompatibility complex on chromosome 17. However, environmental factors also contribute to the development of the disease in the NOD mouse, presumably through controlling the balance between the Th1 and Th2 response in the animal. Recent observations have shown that the NOD mouse has abnormalities in the development of bone marrow-derived antigen-presenting cells. These include the most potent activators of naive T cells, the dendritic cells, which exist in at least two different sub-populations; DC1 cells, responsible for activation of Th1 cells, and DC2 cells, which produce Th2 cells. In addition to activating naïve T cells, the dendritic cells are also involved in generating central and peripheral tolerance to self molecules. In this process DC2 cells appear to be more important for the development of peripheral tolerance than DC1 cells. Besides abnormalities in the development of bone marrow-derived antigen-presenting cells, the NOD mouse also has a defect in the thymic selection of T cells, leading to a higher concentration of autoreactive T cells. We speculate that the NOD mouse may develop an imbalance in the two subsets of dendritic cells with a skewing towards DC1 cells, thus having a reduced ability to generate peripheral tolerance to a number of autoantigens.

Key words: peripheral tolerance; non-obese diabetic mouse; antigen-presenting cells.

Abbreviations used: AIDC – activation-induced cell death, APC – antigen-presenting cells, CSF – colony-stimulating factor, CTL – cytotoxic T lymphocytes, CTS – cataract-prone Shionogi, DC – dendritic cells, GM-CSF – granulocyte macrophage stimulating factor, G0 – agalacto-IgG, IFN – interferon, LCMV – lymphocytic choriomeningitis virus, LPS – lipopolysaccharide, M-CSF – macrophage stimulating factor, MHC – major histocompatibility complex, NOD – non-obese diabetic, PAMP – pathogen-associated molecular pattern, PRR – pattern-recognizing receptor, SDS/PAGE – sodium dodecyl sulfate/ /polyacrylamid gel electrophoresis, TCR – T cell receptor.

A. Górski et al. (eds.), Autoimmunity, 139–160.

1. INDUCTION OF THE IMMUNE RESPONSE

The immune system has evolved to protect the host from invading pathogens. Two general systems of immunity to infectious agents have been selected during evolution: innate or natural immunity, and acquired (adaptive) or specific immunity. Innate immunity refers to the species's basic resistance to infections. It is characterized by a limited ability to distinguish one pathogen from another and it uses families of receptors encoded in the germ line to identify potentially noxious substances. These receptors are referred to as pattern-recognizing receptors (PRRs), which are able to recognise conserved pathogen-associated molecular patterns (PAMPs) associated with microorganisms (Medzhitov and Janeway, 1997a; 1997b). The acquired immunity is characterized by its display of specificity, diversity, memory and self/non-self discrimination. The specificity of the system is a result of its ability to generate a tremendous diversity in its recognition molecules allowing the system to specifically recognize billions of uniquely different structures on foreign antigens. The acquired immune system generates its vast number of antigen-recognizing receptors through the process of somatic gene rearrangement and various means of diversification, which creates random specificities. However, induction of an immune response is only appropriate if the antigen recognized is derived from, or belongs to, a pathogen. Activation of lymphocytes specific for self-antigens, or benign persistent environmental antigens, may result in autoimmune disorders and deleterious hypersensitive reactions, respectively, which is why the imune system's ability to distinguish self from non-self is crucial (Medzhitov and Janeway, 1997a; 1997b). Evidence is now accumulating that the cellular and soluble components of innate immunity provide instructions that enables the acquired immune response to select appropriate antigens and the strategies for their elimination (Fearon and Locksley, 1996). Thus, innate and acquired immunity are closely interlinked, and acquired immunity does not occur independently of innate immunity.

Immunological tolerance, or unresponsiveness, to self-antigens is one of the cornerstones of the aquired immune system, which is why extensive mechanisms have evolved to ensure that effector cells with high specificity for self molecules are eliminated. Tolerance to self is induced by the encounter of immature lymphocytes with self-antigens in the primary lymphoid tissues: the bone marrow in the case of pre-B cells, and the thymus in the case of thymocytes (central tolerance). Once the effector cells are released from the primary lymphoid tissues both the B and T cells may undergo a further selection in the periphery to establish tolerance to antigens not present or not present in sufficient quantities in these primary lymphoid tissues (peripheral tolerance) (Mondino et al., 1996). In the present review we will restrict ourselves to a discussion of T cell immunity/tolerance, as insulin-dependent diabetes is believed to be a T cell-mediated autoimmune disease.

Activation of naive T cells requires two seperate signals in order to induce proliferation. Signal one is received through the antigen receptor (TCR), which recognizes small peptides derived from the proteolytic degradation of polypeptides, presented in complex with major histocompatibility complex (MHC) class I molecules (to $CD8^+$ T cells) or MHC class II molecules (to $CD4^+$ T cells). The second signal is delivered through the co-receptors CD28 (for positive stimulation of the T cells) and CTLA-4 (for down-regulation of the T cell response), which interacts with the co-stimulators CD80 (B7-1) or CD86 (B7-2) expressed on the antigen-presenting cells. A third signal can also be provided via stimulation by various cytokines. If the T cell receives only signal one, it does not become fully activated and may either die through programmed cell death, or apoptosis, or be rendered unresponsive or anergic (Van Parijs et al., 1998).

The co-stimulators CD80 and CD86 are expressed on specialized antigen--presenting cells (APC), such as dendritic cells (DC), macrophages and B cells, which also express MHC class II molecules for activation of $CD4^+$ T cells. Dendritic cells are considered the most potent professional antigen--presenting cells, and although B cells and macrophages might be able to stimulate T cells that have already experienced antigen, the current belief is that only interdigitating DC are able to activate naive $CD4^+$ T (Banchereau and Steinman, 1998; Steinman, 1991). Dendritic cells are, as such, of key importance in ensuring a careful regulation of the $CD4^+$ T cell activation.

Dendritic cells are derived from bone marrow stem cells. They populate the different tissues as immature DC, which are unable to stimulate T cells. The immature DC are characterized by high synthesis but low cell surface expression of MHC class II molecules and low expression of the requisite accessory co-stimulators (Winzler et al., 1997; Young and Steinman, 1996). They are, though, extremely efficient in capturing proteins, which are processed by proteases and loaded onto either MHC class I or MHC class II antigens, depending on the processing and presenting pathway. When DC have captured an antigen and the PRRs expressed on the immature DC interact with a PAMP, a series of events induce the immature DC to differentiate into mature DC (Medzhitov and Janeway, 1997a; 1997b). This maturation is crucial for the initiation of adaptive immunity. A profound change in MHC class II distribution, where the cell surface expression is increased but the synthesis of MHC class II is stopped, characterizes the mature DC. Also, a strong up-regulation of the co-stimulator molecules, induction of integrins and co-receptors, such as LFA-1, and production of various cytokines and chemokines is observed with maturation (Pierre et al., 1997; Winzler et al.,

1997). Mature DC are no longer able of capturing and processing antigen, but are very efficient in presenting antigen. During maturation, the DC migrate into the secondary lymphoid tissue, where they can activate naive T cells expressing T cell receptors specific for antigenic peptides complexed with the MHC class II molecules on the surface of the DC. Many of the antigenic peptides presented by the MHC class II molecules will have originated from self--proteins sampled in the periphery, but the T cells with specificity for these peptides have, in many cases, already either been deleted or have been rendered ignorant by the central tolerance mechanisms.

The T cell response can be characterized as a Th1 or Th2 response, depending on the types of cytokines predominantly synthesized in the activated T cells. Th1 cells secrete IFN-γ, TNF-α and IL-12, while Th2 cells produce IL-4, IL-5 and IL-10 (Kroemer et al., 1996) (Fig. 1). The functional significance of the Th1 and Th2 cell subsets is that their distinct patterns of cytokine secretion lead to strikingly different T cell actions. Th1 cells and

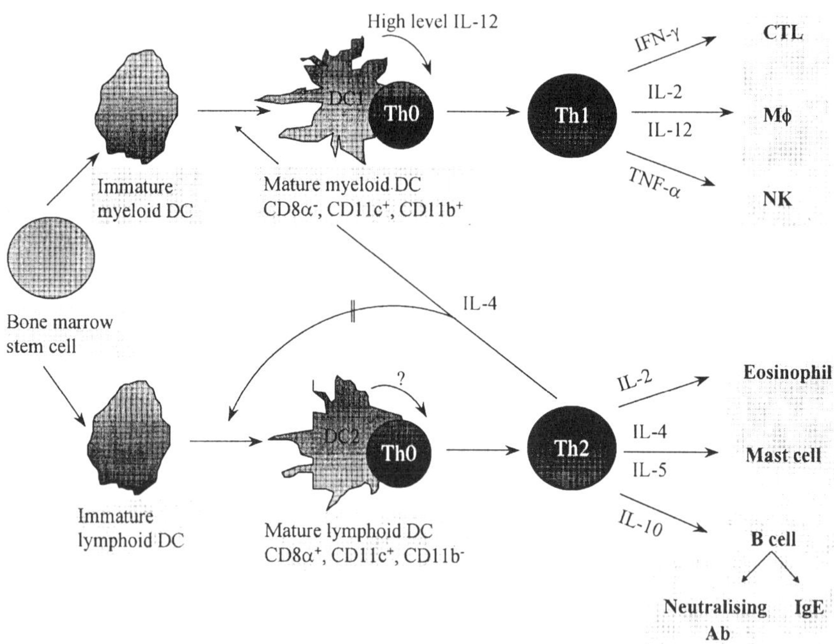

Figure 1. DC1 and DC2 subpopulations provide selective signals to Th0 cells resulting in either Th1 or Th2 immune responses. It is as yet not clear whether the DC subpopulations are derived from different immature DC precursors or immature DC can polarize into mature DC1 or DC2 cells depending on different extracellular signals

their cytokines are the mediators in cellular immune responses, which are characterized by high levels of cytotoxic T lymphocyte (CTL), macrophage and natural killer (NK) cell activation. These cells are thus specialized to eliminate pathogens invading host cells. The Th2 cells are effective stimulators of humoral immune responses, and thus elicit an antibody-mediated reaction that provides protection against extracellular pathogens, such as helminths (Rabinovitch, 1994). The mechanisms determining the differentiation into the two subsets are not fully understood at present, but it seems to rely on signals received very early in the activation process. It is known that the cytokine microenvironment plays an important role in Th0 cell differentiation towards the Th1 or Th2 cell type during immune responses. As DC act as the priming APC for most T cell responses, their role in the differentiation of T cells has now begun to be studied. Rissoan et al. (1999) have recently proposed that the DC not only provide the signals for activation of the T cells, but also the selective signals resulting in either Th1 or Th2 immunity. By sophisticated phenotyping, they characterized two subpopulations of DC from human peripheral blood, which they designated as DC1 and DC2. The DC1 subset was designated as myeloid DCs, and the DC2 subset had a few lymphoid features and did not differentiate into macrophages in response to GM-CSF and M-CSF. Activation of DC1 resulted in the production of a high level of IL-12 and promoted Th1 activation whereas DC2 cells induced Th2 differentiation (Fig. 1). Moreover, it was found that the Th2 cytokine IL-4 enhanced DC1 cell maturation and killed DC2 cells, an effect which was blocked by IFN-γ. Thus, a negative feedback loop from the mature Th cells may selectively inhibit prolonged Th1 or Th2 responses by regulating survival of the appropriate dendritic cell subset. The DC's involvement in the initial commitment of naïve Th cells into the Th1 or Th2 subset has also been explored by Kapsenberg and collegues (1999), who have suggested that the migrating DC carry and additional "signal 3" which biases the naïve Th cell towards either a Th1 or Th2 phenotype.

If an animal is to have a highly specific, yet not self-reacting, immune system, it must in some way be able to tolerate its own antigens. Thus, careful surveillance of the activities of immune cells is necessary to prevent destruction of self tissue. Most individuals do have an immune system able to tolerate or ignore self throughout life. There are, however, some situations where the immune system fails to prevent self-reactions and this can have serious health consequences. Many aspects of autoimmunity and autoimmune diseases have been investigated, but the exact mechanism behind the generation of these complex diseases, i.e. the breakdown of tolerance to self, is still not fully understood. Invading pathogens may share antigenic sequences with peptides derived from self-molecules (antigenic mimicry). If a high T cell response to the foreign peptide is induced, it may break the immunological tolerance or ignorance to self and induce a persistent autoreactive response. Other situations may be related to the way cells in the body are dying. Normally, cells are eliminated in the body through programmed cell death or apoptosis. Mechanisms to eliminate apoptotic cells without causing harm to the individuals have been developed, as, for example, the large number of apoptotic thymocytes in the thymus are cleared out by resident macrophages. However, if cells are particularly stressed or in another way affected, they may die abnormally by necrosis. This releases a range of intracellular molecules, notably molecules such as RNA and DNA, heat shock proteins and other stress molecules (Gallucci et al., 1999). These molecules are not normally available to the immune system and, because there is an extensive sequence conservation of these molecules from pathogens to animals and because they are potent activators of dendritic cells, their release may elicit an autoimmune response. Many autoimmune diseases are T cell-mediated, and several studies indicate that a functional imbalance between the two Th cell subsets is a key determinant in establishing autoimmune pathology (Kroemer et al., 1996; Rabinovitch, 1994).

Type 1 (insulin-dependent) diabetes mellitus is an example of a chronic organ-specific autoimmune disease attacking the insulin-producing cells in the pancreas, resulting in insulin deficiency. As a relatively common disease, type 1 diabetes mellitus has been extensively studied. Even so the triggering of the breakdown in tolerance, or the mechanism through which, this occurs, is still not understood, and much less information is available on the etiology of the disease than on the pathogenesis. We will here use a spontaneous mouse model for type 1 diabetes, the non-obese diabetic (NOD) mouse, to argue that one of the contributing factors for the disease progression is the inability to induce normal or sufficient peripheral tolerance.

2. PATHOGENICITY OF DIABETES IN THE NOD MOUSE

The NOD mouse is a spontaneous model for human type 1 (insulin-dependent) diabetes mellitus. The NOD mouse was derived from a cataract mouse found among outbred Jcl: ICR mice in 1966. During inbreeding and selection of the cataract-prone phenotype resulting in the cataract-prone Shionogi (CTS) strain, a female mouse with diabetic signs as observed and used to establish the NOD strain in 1980 (Makino et al., 1980) (Fig. 2). As in human type 1 diabetics, the disease in the NOD mouse appears to be a chronic autoimmune disease characterized by a lymphocytic infiltration of the islets

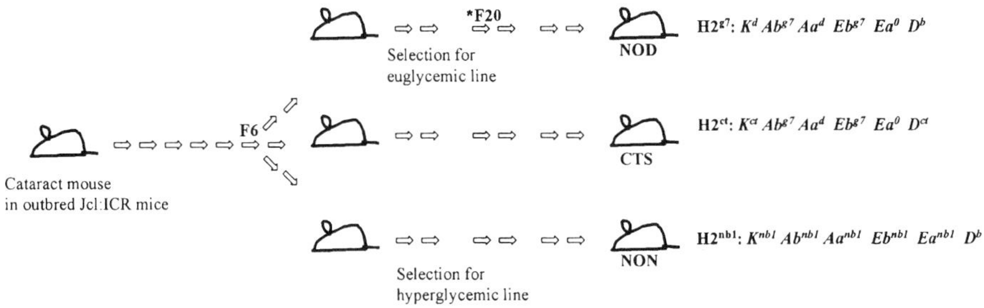

Figure 2. The genotype of the NOD mouse and its related lines. The NOD mouse was derived from a cataract mouse identified among Jcl: ICR outbred mice, which was used to develop an inbred cataract-prone strain, the CTS mouse (cataract Shionogi): During the breeding, two sublines were separated at the 6th generation selected for development of euglycemic and hyperglycemic phenotype. At the 20th generation (*F20) a diabetic female mouse of the euglycemic line was identified and used to establish the NOD mouse (Makino et al., 1980)

of pancreas, production of a number of autoantibodies with islet-reactivity and, finally, a selective destruction of the insulin-producing β cells in the pancreas. The lymphocytic infiltration starts as early as 3–6 weeks of age (Gazda et al., 1997; Katz et al., 1993) with an initial influx of DC and macrophages, which are later followed by T and B cells (Jansen et al., 1994). The lymphocytic inflammation consists initially of peri-islet located lymphocytes, which are not activated and remain benign for a long time. However, at 10 to 14 weeks of age, β cell-specific $CD4^+$ and $CD8^+$ T cells become activated and, within 3 weeks, they destroy a sufficient number of insulin-producing β cells to cause clinical diabetes. Depending on environmental factors, the incidence of diabetes in a typical high-incidence colony is between 80–90% in females and 40–50% in males by 30 weeks of age. The switch from benign to malignant autoimmunity in the NOD mice appears to be central to the disease progression in the NOD mouse. This, as yet unexplainable, switch from benign to malignant infiltration of the islets has also been observed in the BDC2.5 T cell receptor transgenic NOD mouse (Katz et al., 1993), which expresses on most of its T cells the rearranged T cell receptor genes isolated from a diabetogenic CTL line. Although a massive intra-islet inflammation of T cells is seen from 3 weeks of age in the transgenic NOD mice, they do not develop diabetes until 10–25 weeks of age, much like the pattern of diabetes onset in the control NOD mice.

The T cells play a crucial role in the development of diabetes in the NOD mouse. Many experiments have shown that T cells isolated from diabetic females can accelerate the onset of diabetes if injected into irradiated non-diabetic NOD mice (Wicker et al., 1986). Th1 cells are believed to be the primary $CD4^+$ T cells mediating type 1 diabetes, and, indeed, β cell-specific

T cell clones that exhibit a Th1 phenotype have been found to efficiently transfer diabetes in NOD (Trembleau et al., 1999). However, such transfer studies have also shown that both $CD4^+$ and $CD8^+$ cells are required for the development of diabetes in the recipient mice. Moreover, it has been shown that depleting young animals of DC and macrophages prevents insulitis and diabetes (Hutchings et al., 1990), demonstrating an important role for these cells in the onset of the autoimmune disease in the NOD mouse.

Autoantibodies to many of the same islet-derived antigens observed in humans have also been found in the NOD mouse (Pontesilli et al., 1987; Ziegler et al., 1989). We have compared insulin-specific autoantibodies in non-diabetic and diabetic NOD mice with control mice and found no difference in the isotype or concentration of the insulin-specific Ig. Where we did find a difference was in the concentration of insulin-specific agalacto-IgGs (G0s), which sharply increased from 12 weeks and onwards in the NOD mice compared with control mice (Malling et al., unpublished observations). Agalacto-IgG does not have terminal galactose in the N-linked oligosaccharide chain in the Fc region. Although this glycosylation modification is naturally occurring, the relative level of G0 antibodies in systemic autoimmune diseases such as rheumatoid arthritis (RA) and systemic lupus erythematosus (SLE) is higher than seen in age- and sex-matched normal controls (recently reviewed by Delves (1998)). Using a collagen-induced arthritis model, Rademacher et al. (1994) showed that *in vitro* produced G0-antibodies specific for collagen can be pathogenic. It was interesting to note that the increase in the G0 of the insulin-autoantibodies in the NOD mice coincided in time with the shift from benign to malignant autoimmunity. Any link between these two events has yet to be established, though.

The role of autoantibodies in the development of diabetes has not been fully explored. There is no evidence that these autoantibodies are pathogenic, and the disease cannot be transferred by serum from affected subjects (Serreze et al., 1998). However, the absence of B cells in the NOD mice prevents the development or at least significantly delays the onset of diabetes. This has been demonstrated by crossing the $Ig\mu^{0/0}$ mutation onto the NOD background to create congenic NOD.Ig$\mu^{0/0}$ mice that do not produce B cells due to a lack of B cell receptors (Serreze et al., 1996). These mice do not become diabetic at the normal incidence rate. The protective effect of $Ig\mu^{0/0}$ has been interpreted as if the B cells function as antigen-presenting cells for naïve T cells, because injection of antibodies from diabetic NOD mice into NOD.Ig$\mu^{0/0}$ mice does not induce diabetes in the recipient mice (Serreze et al., 1998). It cannot be excluded, however, that autoantibodies have more than a pedestrian function in the development of diabetes in mice and humans.

3. GENETIC PREDISPOSITION

As in humans, the disease in the NOD mouse is determined by several genes (*Idd1-19*) (Table 1). At least three of these genes have been linked to the MHC region, whilst the non-MHC genes map to other chromosomes (Serreze and Leiter, 1994; Wicker et al., 1995). The non-MHC genes are collectively responsible for the autoimmune-susceptible genotype of the animals, whereas the H2 alleles determine the predominant feature of the autoimmune disease. This can be demonstrated by the fact that the congenic NOD.H2^{b} (K^b A^b E^b D^b) mouse does not develop diabetes but is a model for the autoimmune Sjögren' disease, and NOD.H2^{h4} (K^k A^k E^k D^k) mouse spontaneously develops thyroditis but not diabetes (Wicker, 1997). The MHC class II molecules especially are a key components in the development of diabetes, and the homozygosity of the class II genes have been shown necessary for disease susceptibility.

The MHC-linked diabetogenic genes collectively contribute 42% to the familial clustering of diabetes in the NOD mouse (Todd et al., 1987). The NOD mouse has a unique MHC haplotype: K^d Ab^{g7} Aa^d Eb^{g7} Ea^0 and D^b (Fig. 2). The only MHC class II restriction element expressed in the mouse, I-A, has an unusual structure, with a histidine and a serine in positions Aβ56 and

Table 1. Chromosomal localization of the *Idd* loci

Locus	Adjacent gene(s)	Chromosome	cM position
Idd1	MHC	17	19.5
Idd2	*Ncam*	9	22.0
Idd3	*Fgf2*	3	19.2
Idd4	*Nf1*	4	44.0
Idd5	*Fn1/Pax3*	5	40.0
Idd6		7	syntenic
Idd7	*Sle*	7	4.0
Idd8	*Tcra*	14	3.5
Idd9	*Elp1*	4	82.0
Idd10	*Tshb/Amy1*	3	48.5
Idd11	*Ssdh1*	11	64.6
Idd12	*Glud/Tcra*	14	12.0
Idd13	*Il1*	2	71.0
Idd14		5	syntenic
Idd16	MHC, *Tnfa*	17	18.0
Idd17	*Glrb, Fgg*	3	39.0
Idd18	*Amy1, Egf*	3	56.3
Idd19	*Raf1*	6	57.5

Further information can be found at
http://www.informatics.jax.org//searches/markerfrom.shtml

Aβ57, where most other Aβ subunits encode a proline and an aspartic acid, respectively. Construction of NOD mice containing transgenes encoding mutated and different MHC alleles have shown that the unusual structure of the ab^{g7} (Lund et al., 1990; Quartely-Papafio et al., 1995) and the lack of I-E expression (Lund et al., 1990; Nishimoto et al., 1987) are critical for the diabetogenic phenotype and consistent with the involvement of $CD4^{+}$ cells in the autoimmune phenotype. The mutated Ab^{g7} and the Ea^{d} transgenes appear to protect the NOD from developing diabetes through different mechanisms. Thus, peri-islet infiltration of T cells, but no switch to malignant infiltration, was observed in the NOD.Ab^{g7}-Pro56 and NOD.Ab^{g7}-Asp (Trembleau et al., 1999) transgenic mice, while restoring the expression of I-E with a functional Ea^{d} gene completely abrogated all signs of autoimmunity (Lund et al., 1990; Nishimoto et al., 1987). In addition, either the structure or the expression of MHC class I alleles may also be important for the diabetogenic phenotype, because introducing $H2\text{-}L^{d}$ as a transgene back-crossed into the NOD protects against development of diabetes (Miyazaki et al., 1992). This protection could, though, also be derived from the genomic region flanking the transgene co-introduced into the NOD mice through the back-crossing.

At least four additional MHC-linked diabetogenic genes exist in the NOD mouse besides the MHC class I and class II alleles. Analysis of congenic intra-MHC recombinant NOD mice, where a >6.6 cM region centromeric to *Lpm2* in the NOD mouse was replaced with the similar region derived from a B10.A(R209) mouse, showed that this region protects the animals from developing both insulitis and diabetes (Hattori et al., 1999), even though these mice have the rest of the MHC region of the NOD mouse. More refined dissection of the region suggests that at least 3 diabetogenic genes map to this region. Furthermore, construction of congenic NOD.$H2^{ct}$ containing the MHC region of the CTS mouse (Fig. 2), which shares the MHC class II alleles with the NOD mouse, has demonstrated that there exists at least one additional diabetogenic gene (*Idd16*) (Ikegami et al., 1995), possibly located in the MHC class III region (Lund et al., 1993). The phenotype of these four MHC-linked diabetogenic genes has yet to be established.

4. ENVIRONMENTAL FACTORS

The disease in type 1 diabetes mellitus is genetically complex, and several susceptibility and protective genes have been identified in both human diabetes and in animal models of the disease. However, the concordance rate in monozygotic twins is only about 50%, and the large differences in diabetes incidence between colonies of NOD mice indicates that the determination of type 1 diabetes is multifactorial, with a number of as yet unidentified environmental factors contributing to the disease. Some of the environmental factors known to influence the development of diabetes in NOD mice include diet, viral infection and exposure to microbial agents and temperature (see Rabinovitch, 1994 for review). Studies have shown that NOD mice kept on an essential fatty acid-deficient diet or a diet where chloroform-soluble components have been removed have a significantly reduced cumulative incidence of diabetes without affecting the insulitis process (Benhamou et al., 1995; Coleman et al., 1990). A viral origin of diabetes was one of the first etiological hypotheses, but, intriguingly, it has been shown that NOD animals raised in a pathogen-free environment have an increased incidence (>90%) of disease, suggesting that certain pathogenic infections can reduce or prevent the onset of the disease. Direct infections with a number of viruses can also prevent diabetes in the NOD mice (see Rabinovitch, 1994 for review). In addition, immunisation protocols with adjuvants containing microbacterial extracts will induce protection from disease in the NOD mice (Rabinovitch, 1994; Serreze and Leiter, 1994). Finally, induction of stress has also been shown to induce protection against development of diabetes in the animals (Saravia-Fernandez et al., 1996). It thus seems that a general activation of the immune system and up-regulation of APC function will protect the susceptible animals from developing type 1 diabetes.

The mechanisms responsible for the effects the environmental factors have on the onset of diabetes in the NOD mouse have yet to be determined. However, there are strong indications that their influence on the disease may be caused by a shift in the balance between a Th1 and Th2 response. If the autoreactive immune response in autoimmune-prone individuals is initiated as a Th1 type, it will progress to a full-blown disease, whereas a general shift in the cytokine balance towards a Th2 response prevents the autoimmune disease. The onset of diabetes in NOD mice, which are deficient in IL-4, can, for example, be prevented by IL-4 injections (Rapoport et al., 1993), strongly suggesting that a Th2 response protects against development of diabetes.

5. AUTOREACTIVITY

Several studies have shown that the NOD mouse has a defect in the thymic selection of T cells, leading to a higher concentration of autoreactive T cells released into the periphery (De Luca et al., 1995; Kanagawa et al., 1998). Ridgway et al. (1998) likewise proposed that the disease susceptibility in the NOD mouse could be explained by an inefficient negative selection of T cells in the thymus and that this was caused by the I-A^{g7} molecules. They immunised NOD mice, congenic NOD.H2^{h4} mice (H2 haplotype: K^k A^k E^k

D^k), NOD-Ab^k transgenic mice (homozygous for I-A^{g7} but also expressing I-A$^{k/d}$ molecule) and congenic B10.H2^{g7} (containing the MHC region of the NOD mouse on a C56BL/10 background) with different self peptides mixed with complete Freund's adjuvant. They then examined the lymph nodes for the presence of autoreactive CD4$^+$ cells, i.e., CD4$^+$ T cells able to proliferate in response to APC expressing the appropriate self-antigens. They found that NOD mice homozygous for I-A^{g7} did elicit proliferation of autoreactive T cells irrespective of whether the I-A^k transgene was expressed or not, but that (NOD×NOD.H2^{h4}) F1 mice heterozygous for I-A^{g7} failed to induce autoreactive CD4$^+$ cells. Neither the congenic NOD.H2^{h4} nor B10. H2^{g7} mice were able to elicit detectable levels of autoreactive CD4$^+$ cells, demonstrating that homozygous I-A^{g7} is necessary but not sufficient for inducing proliferation of autoreactive T cell clones.

In an attempt to understand the lack of tolerance induction in the NOD mouse, we made a study on DC derived from bone marrow of NOD, NOD.H2^{h4} and control CBA mice. We found that both the NOD and the NOD.H2^{h4} dendritic cells expressed significantly less MHC class II on their surface as well as both of the co-stimulator molecules CD80 and CD86. The number of cells expressing MHC class II and CD80/86 as well as the number of molecules per cell were greatly decreased compared with those on dendritic cells from non-autoimmune CBA mice. These findings correlated with the failure of these dendritic cells to induce T cell proliferation in an antigen--dependent manner (Strid et al., Clin. Exp. Immunol., in press).

The crystal structures of MHC class II molecules have shown that the relatively well-conserved aspartic acid residue at position Ab57 forms a salt bridge with residue Arg76 on the α-helix of Aa to stabilize the peptide-binding groove. The serine at position 57 of the Ab^{g7} prevents formation of this salt bridge, giving I-A^{g7} an intrinsic instability characterized by the formation of a high fraction of unstable molecules in SDS/PAGE analysis. This makes the MHC class II molecules poor binders of peptides with weak affinities for and fast dissociation rates of the peptides (Carrasco-Marin et al., 1996). In addition, the I-A^{g7} molecule has a short half-life on APC (Carrasco-Marin et al., 1996).

According to the avidity model of the thymic selection of T cells, it is not the intrinsic affinity of the TCR for its ligand alone which determines the faith of the thymocytes, but the avidity of the interaction between the thymocyte and the APC defined as the combination of the intrinsic TCR affinity, the density of the TCR on the thymocytes, the density of the peptide: MHC ligand on the thymic DC and the potency of the costimulatory signalling. The fact that I-A^{g7} is a poor peptide binder and may be expressed at a lower concentration on the APC in the thymus would thus have a far-reaching effect on thymic selection by dramatically decreasing the effective dose of I-A^{g7}: self-

-peptides on the selecting DC surface. The net result of a low dose of MHC: peptide complex would be an increase in TCR affinity to achieve an equivalent avidity threshold for positive and negative selection. This would result in the selection of a population of high-affinity, self-reactive and potentially autoreactive T cells.

6. DEFECTS IN BONE MARROW-DERIVED CELLS

There is increasing evidence for abnormalities in bone marrow-derived cells in diabetics. Langmuir et al. (1993) showed that NOD mice are somewhat deficient in their *in vitro* response to IL-3, GM-CSF and IL-5. They found that fewer progeny cells were produced *in vitro* from bone marrow cell suspensions in response to increasing concentrations of the growth factors compared with bone marrow cells derived from the non-diabetic BALB/c mice. Looking at the cytokines produced by the APCs, we (Strid and Lund, unpublished results) and others (Serreze et al., 1993a) have not found any difference in TNF-α production between LPS-stimulated peritoneal macrophages from NOD and diabetes-resistant control strains, which contrasts with the findings of Jacob et al. (1990; 1996). Nor did we find any differences in the cytokine profiles between LPS-stimulated bone marrow-derived dendritic cells from NOD and control mice (Strid et al., in press). However, LPS--stimulated macrophages from the NOD mouse are known to be poor IL-1 producers (Jacob et al., 1990; 1996; Serreze et al., 1993a), suggesting that at least some macrophages in the NOD mouse are not fully differentiated. Indeed, Serreze et al. (1993a; 1993b) found a defect in the development of macrophages from NOD bone marrow cell suspensions in response to CSF-1 *in vitro*. These NOD-derived CSF-1-generated macrophages showed a functional deficiency, where the MHC class I expression was aberrantly down-regulated in response to IFN-γ, while MHC class I expression on macrophages derived similarly from C57BL/KsJ mice remained on the same level after IFN-γ treatment (Serreze et al., 1993b). In addition, the bone marrow-derived NOD macrophages required the presence of both CSF-1 and IFN-γ to induce expression of significant levels of the receptor for CSF-1, the *c-fms* proto--oncogen. In contrast, macrophages from diabetes-resistant control mice expressed high levels of *c-fgm* in response to CSF-1 only, and macrophages from the non-obese non-diabetic NON mice down-regulated the expression of *c-fgm* when incubated with both CSF-1 and IFN-γ. The NOD macrophages also had an abnormal regulation of the IFN-γ receptor, *Ifgr* (Serreze et al., 1993a). The difference between NOD and control mice was observed as differences in the mRNA levels, which may be caused by a reduced activity of protein kinase C in the NOD macrophages (Serreze et al., 1993a). The developmental abnormalities in the cytokine-stimulated macrophages in the NOD mouse are controlled by non-MHC linked diabetogenic genes (Serreze et al., 1993b).

It is now widely accepted that the dendritic cells are the most important and potent professional APC. Even so not much work has been published on dendritic cells in the NOD mouse. We have, however, recently described that the development of DC, as that of macrophages, in the NOD mice is abnormal compared to that of DC derived form diabetes-resistant control strains. As mentioned previously, we found that myeloid DC generated by cultivating bone marrow stem cells in the presence of GM-CSF expressed very low levels of MHC class II molecules and the co-receptors CD80 and CD86 on the cell surface even following activation with both LPS and IFN-γ. In addition, we could not induce IL-2 production in T cells in an antigen-specific manner (Strid et al., submitted for publication). Bone marrow-derived DC from the congenic NOD.H2^{h4} (K^k, A^k, E^k, D^k) mouse also failed to express MHC class II, CD80/CD86 and to stimulate T cell proliferation, suggesting that, like the defective development of macrophages, the differentiation abnormalities of dendritic cells in the NOD mice are not controlled by genes located in the MHC region (Strid et al., in press).

An abnormal development in the production of dendritic cells appears to be associated with diabetes also in the other spontaneous model for type 1 diabetes; the BB-DP rat. A lower number of dendritic cells could be isolated from the BB-DP rat compared with non-diabetic Wistar rats. The DC had the same immature phenotype as we have described for the NOD mouse, with low MHC class II and co-receptor expression and an inability to elicit an allo--MLR response *in vitro* (Delemarre et al., 1999). Even human diabetics appear to have a defect in the development of DC. Takahashi et al. (1998) obtained a lower yield of DC in response to GM-CSF and IL-4 from adherent peripheral blood cells from diabetic patients compared with age-, sex- and MHC class II-matched non-diabetic controls. In addition the *in vitro*-derived DC from the diabetic patients showed a reduced expression of the co-receptors CD80 and CD86 as well as a lower stimulation of autologous CD4$^+$ T cells compared with dendritic cells derived from the non-diabetic controls.

The abnormalities in the development of myeloid DC in type 1 diabetic humans and in the spontaneous animal models for type 1 diabetes do not seem to render them unable to elicit an immune response. There are no indications that type 1 diabetics are immunologically incompetent. The apparent immaturity of diabetic DC may, however, suggest that there is a linkage between the abnormal production of certain bone marrow-derived hematopoietic cells and the ability to induce self-tolerance.

7. IS THERE AN IMBALANCE IN THE DEVELOPMENT OF DC IN DIABETICS AND CAN THIS EXPLAIN THE LACK OF SELF-TOLERANCE IN THESE PATIENTS?

Peripheral tolerance is the mechanism which maintains unresponsiveness to antigens that are present only in peripheral tissues and not in the generative lymphoid organs. Peripheral mechanisms may also inactivate or kill lymphocytes that are specific for ubiquitous self-antigens but which escaped central tolerance, for any reason. Tolerance in $CD4^+$ T lymphocytes may be induced either by a process of functional inactivation (anergy) or by apoptotic cell death as a result of antigen stimulation (activation-induced cell death, AICD). It is also possible that the functions of $CD4^+$ T cells are suppressed by other suppressive lymphocytes. The consequence of antigen recognition, i.e. activation or tolerance, depends mainly on two factors: how the antigen is presented to lymphocytes (the nature of the APC, concentration of the antigen, tissue location and persistence of the antigen), and how the responses of specific lymphocytes to that antigen are regulated. Recognition of self antigen in peripheral lymphoid tissues is a normal phenomenon, but pathological autoimmunity should be prevented by controlling what happens to lymphocytes after they respond to self-peptides. Since DC are likely to be the activators of most T cell responses, it does not seem unreasonable to believe that DC play an important role in the induction of peripheral tolerance as well as central tolerance.

The autoimmune response in the NOD mouse appears to consist of two seperate events. First, there is a benign infiltration into important endocrine organs, such as the islet of Langerhans, which starts very early in life. Even if the animal expresses predominantly β cell-reactive $CD8^+$ T cells, no tissue damage is seen during this phase. However, at 10 weeks or later, an autoreactive immune response is initiated in the majority of the female and, depending on the environment, also in a fraction of the male mice, which very rapidly leads to destruction of the insulin-producing cells. It has yet to be established what precipitates this malignant autoimmune response. But why do not all the animals become diabetics, and why does an induction of Th2 responses in the animals appear to protect against development of type I diabetes? We hypothesize that the spontaneous development of autoimmune disease(s) in the NOD mouse relates to a failure of peripheral tolerance induction. This is supported by the experiments of Clare-Salzler et al. (1992), who reported that transfer of DC derived from the pancreatic lymph node of NOD mice, but not from any other lymph nodes, protected against development of diabetes, suggesting that an increase in the capacity to induce peripheral tolerance will protect against development of the autoimmune disease. The insufficient induction of peripheral tolerance, as hypothesized, in unrelated to the MHC alleles of the NOD mouse, since NOD.H2^{h4} congenic mice spontaneously develop autoimmune thyroditis if fed iodine in their drinking water.

Pulendran et al. (1997) demonstrated that two distinct DC subtypes could be differentially expanded in mice *in vivo*. Treatment of the animals with GM--CSF *in vivo* preferentially expanded a DC subset with features characteristic of DC2 cells, which have the ability to activate naïve CD4^{+} T cells into a Th2 type. In contrast, mice injected with the cytokine Flt-3 ligand (Maraskovsky et al., 1996; Pulendran et al., 1997) dramatically expanded a different subset of DC with high expression of IL-12 and IFN-γ (Pulendran et al., 1999). The Flt-3 ligand-treated mice produced a high level of Th1 cells and, if immunised with ovalbumin, they predominantly produced IgG2a antibodies, whereas GM-CSF-treated mice immunised with ovalbumin predominately elicited an IgG1 antibody response. Pulendran and colleagues (1998) have previously shown that mice treated with Flt-3 ligand had a dramatically enhanced sensitivity of antigen-specific B and T cell responses and that the Flt-3-treated mice could elicit a productive immune response to otherwise tolerogenic protocols.

Human diabetics and the two spontaneous animal models for type 1 diabetes, the BB-DP rat and the NOD mouse, share a defect in the development of DC. Fewer monocytes cells are produced from primary (bone marrow) and secondary (spleen) lymphoid cell suspensions or from peripheral blood cells in response to various growth factors (GM-CSF, M-CSF, IL-3, IL-5) relative to appropriate non-diabetic controls (Delemarre et al., 1999; Langmuir et al., 1993; Takahashi et al., 1998). In addition, at least in the case of the animal models, the GM-CSF-generated dendritic cells appear to be developmentally arrested at a precursor state, with little or no MHC class II and CD80/CD86 cell surface expression (Strid et al., in press) (Delemarre et al., 1999). The GM-CSF-generated DC from the NOD mouse also proved to produce a very limited amount of IL-12 in response to LPS and IFN-γ compared with non--autoimmune controls, indicating that they may be of the DC2 subset (Strid et al., in press). This abnormal developmental response to GM-CSF could affect the balance of the DC1/DC2 subset in the autoimmune-prone animals or individuals both in the primary and secondary lymphoid tissues as well as in the periphery. A deficient maturation of the DC2s in the autoimmune-susceptible animals or individuals could polarize the DC population towards a predominant DC1 subset. If the observation of Pulendran et al. (1997; 1999), that the DC1s are less able to induce central and peripheral tolerance in the host, is correct, the individuals with a predominant DC1 population may be more prone to developing autoimmune diseases. In addition, a skewing towards a DC1 response to self-antigens would shift the T cell response from a non-destructive Th2 to the destructive Th1 response prevailing in the animals or individuals that develop diabetes.

Although a lack of centrally and peripherally induced tolerance/ignorance to self proteins contributes to the development of the disease in the NOD mouse, it cannot explain the shift from benign to malign autoimmunity in the mice. A number of transgenic models have been explored to search for explanations for insulin-dependent diabetes. In these mice, foreign transgenes, LCMB gp120 (Ohashi et al., 1991; Oldstone et al., 1991) or membrane-attached ovalbumin (Kurts et al., 1997a; 1997b), were put under the control of the rat insulin promoter (RIP) and microinjected into C56BL/6 embryos in order to direct the expression to the insulin-producing cells in the pancreas. One of the transgenic lines also expressed the transgene in the thymus (Oldstone et al., 1991), whereas no presence of transgenic mRNA could be detected in the thymus of the two other transgenic lines (Kurts et al., 1997b; Ohashi et al., 1991). Despite this, central tolerance against the transgene could be observed, as the ovalbumin transgenic mice, when crossed with transgenic mice expressing an ovalbumin-specific H2-K^b-restricted T cell receptor, showed a significant deletion of the antigen-specific T cells (Kurts et al., 1997b). The lessons from these 3 transgenic mouse lines were that, although the transgene was predominantly expressed in the insulin-producing β cells, the whole T cell population appeared ignorant towards the antigen, i.e., the induction of peripheral tolerance was adequate to regulate the T cell population. If the animals were infected with LCMV, however, β cell destruction was observed within weeks, and the autoimmune response could be transferred with $CD4^+$ and $CD8^+$ T cells to non-infected transgenic mice (Ohashi et al., 1991; Oldstone et al., 1991). Autoimmune destruction was observed to require a threshold level of antigen--specific T cells (Kurts et al., 1997a; 1997b) and, although $CD8^+$ T cells alone would be able to induce autoimmune disease in the animals upon transfer, the threshold level was much higher than in the presence of antigen-specific $CD4^+$ T cells (Kurts et al., 1997a).

Extending this discussion to the NOD mouse, which spontaneously develops diabetes, one may presume that, around week 12, a number of β cells will suddenly be destroyed and numerous intra-cellular proteins released and captured by DC. The dendritic cells will migrate to the draining lymph node, where they will present the self antigen to T cells and elicit an autoimmune response. Because of the unfavourable balance in DC1/DC2 cells, the threshold level of activated β cell-specific T cells required for mounting a full-blown autoimmune response is much lower than in non-diabetic control animals.

Acknowledgment. This work has been supported by grants from The British Diabetic Association, The Arthritis and Rheumatism Council and The Wellcome Trust.

REFERENCES

Banchereau J. and Steinman R. M. (1998): Dendritic cells and the control of immunity. Nature, **392**, 245–252.

Benhamou P. Y., Mullen Y., Clare-Salzler M., Sangkharat A., Benhamou C., Shevlin L. and Go V. L. (1995): Essential fatty acid deficiency prevents autoimmune diabetes in nonobese diabetic mice through a positive impact on antigen-presenting cells and Th2 lymphocytes. Pancreas, **11**, 26–37.

Carrasco-Marin E., Shimizu J., Kanagawa O. and Unanue E. R. (1996): The class II MHC I-A^{g7} molecules from non-obese diabetic mice are poor peptide binders. J. Immunol., **156**, 450–458.

Clare-Salzler M. J., Brooks J., Chai A., Vanherle K. and Anderson C. (1992): Prevention of diabetes in non-obese diabetic mice by dendritic cell transfer. J. Clin. Invest., **90**, 741–748.

Coleman D. L., Kuzava J. E. and Leiter E. H. (1990): Effect of diet on incidence of diabetes in non-obese diabetic mice. Diabetes, **39**, 432–436.

Delemarre F. G., Simons P. J., de Heer H. J. and Drexhage H. A. (1999): Signs of immaturity of splenic dendritic cells from the autoimmune prone biobreeding rat: consequences for the *in vitro* expansion of regulator and effector T cells. J. Immunol., **162**, 1795–1801.

De Luca D., Bluestone J. A., Shultz L. D., Sharrow S. O. and Tatsumi Y. (1995): Programmed differentiation of murine thymocytes during fetal thymus organ culture. J. Immunol. Methods, **178**, 13–29.

Delves P. J. (1998): The role of glycosylation in autoimmune disease. Autoimmunity, **27**, 239–253.

Fearon D. T. and Locksley R. M. (1996): The instructive role of innate immunity in the acquired immune response. Science, **272**, 50–54.

Gallucci S., Lolkema M. and Matzinger P. (1999): Natural adjuvants: endogenous activators of dendritic cells. Nat. Med., **5**, 1249–1255.

Gazda L. S., Charlton B. and Lafferty K. J. (1997): Diabetes results from a late change in the autoimmune response of NOD mice. J. Autoimmun., **10**, 261–270.

Hattori M., Yamato E., Itoh N., Senpuku H., Fujisawa T., Yoshino M., Fukuda M., Matsumoto E., Toyonaga T., Nakagawa I., Petruzzelli M., McMurray A., Weiner H., Sagai T., Moriwaki K., Shiroishi T., Maron R. and Lund T. (1999): Cutting edge: Homologous recombination of the MHC class I K region defines new MHC-linked diabetogenic susceptibility gene(s) in non-obese diabetic mice. J. Immunol., **163**, 1721–1724.

Hutchings P., Rosen H., O'Reilly L., Simpson E., Gordon S. and Cooke A. (1990): Transfer of diabetes in mice prevented by blockade of adhesion-promoting receptor on macrophages. Nature, **348**, 639–642.

Ikegami H., Makino S., Yamato E., Kawaguchi Y., Ueda H., Sakamoto T., Takekawa K. and Ogihara T. (1995): Identification of a new susceptibility locus for insulin-dependent diabetes-mellitus by ancestral haplotype congenic mapping. J. Clin. Invest., **96**, 1936–1942.

Jacob C. O., Aiso S., Michie S. A., McDevitt H. O. and Acha O. H. (1990): Prevention of diabetes in non-obese diabetic mice by tumor necrosis factor (TNF): similarities between TNF--alpha and interleukin 1. Proc. Natl. Acad. Sci. USA, **87**, 968–972.

Jacob C. O., Lee S. K. and Strassman G. (1996): Mutational analysis of TNF-alpha gene reveals a regulatory role for the 3'-untranslated region in the genetic predisposition to lupus-like autoimmune disease. J. Immunol., **156**, 3043–3050.

Jansen A., Homodelarche F., Hooijkaas H., Leenen P. J., Dardenne M. and Drexhage H. A. (1994): Immunohistochemical characterization of monocytes-macrophages and dendritic cells involved in the initiation of the insulitis and beta-cell destruction in NOD mice. Diabetes, **43**, 667–675.

Kanagawa O., Martin S. M., Vaupel B. A., Carrasco-Marin E. and Unanue E. R. (1998): Autoreactivity of T cells from non-obese diabetic mice: An I-A^{g7}-dependent reaction. Proc. Natl. Acad. Sci. USA, **95**, 1721–1724.

Kapsenberg M. L., Hilkens C. M., Wierenga E. A. and Kalinski P. (1999): The paradigm of type 1 and type 2 antigen-presenting cells. Implications for atopic allergy. Clin. Exp. Allergy, **29** (suppl. 2), 33–36.

Katz J. D., Wang B., Haskins K., Benoist C. and Mathis D. (1993): Following a diabetogenic T cell from genesis through pathogenesis. Cell, **74**, 1089–1100.

Kroemer G., Hirsch F., Gonzalez-Garcia A. and Martinez C. (1996): Differential involvement of Th1 and Th2 cytokines in autoimmune diseases. Autoimmunity, **24**, 25–33.

Kurts C., Carbone F. R., Barnden M., Blanas E., Allison J., Heath W. R. and Miller J. F. (1997a): $CD4^+$ T cell help impairs $CD8^+$ T cell deletion induced by cross-presentation of self--antigens and favors autoimmunity. J. Exp. Med., **186**, 2057–2062.

Kurts C., Kosaka H., Carbone F. R., Miller J. F. and Heath W. R. (1997b): Class I-restricted cross-presentation of exogenous self-antigens leads to deletion of autoreactive $CD8^+$ T cells. J. Exp. Med., **186**, 239–245.

Langmuir P. B., Bridgett M. M., Bothwell A. L. M. and Crispe I. N. (1993): Bone-marrow abnormalities in the non-obese diabetic mouse. Int. Immunol., **5**, 169–177.

Lund T., O'Reilly L., Hutchings P., Kanagawa O., Simpson E., Gravely R., Chandler P., Dyson J., Picard J. K., Edwards A., Kioussis D. and Cooke A. (1990): Prevention of insulin-dependent diabetes mellitus in non-obese diabetic mice by transgenes encoding modified I-A β-chain or normal I-E α-chain. Nature, **345**, 727–729.

Lund T., Shaikh S., Kendall E., Campbell R. D., Hattori M., Makino S. and Cooke A. (1993): RFLP analysis of the MHC class III region defines unique haplotypes for the non-obese diabetic, cataract Shionogi and the non-obese non-diabetic mouse strains. Diabetologia, **36**, 727–733.

Makino S., Kunimoto K., Muraoka Y., Mizushima Y., Katagiri K. and Tochino Y. (1980): Breeding of a non-obese, diabetic strain of mice. Jikken Dobutsu, **29**, 1–13.

Maraskovsky E., Brasel K., Teepe M., Roux E. R., Lyman S. D., Shortman K. and McKenna H. J. (1996): Dramatic increase in the numbers of functionally mature dendritic cells in Flt3 ligand-treated mice: multiple dendritic cell subpopulations identified. J. Exp. Med., **184**, 1953–1962.

Medzhitov R. and Janeway C. A. Jr. (1997a): Innate immunity: the virtues of a nonclonal system of recognition. Cell, **91**, 295–298.

Medzhitov R. and Janeway C. A. Jr. (1997b): Innate immunity: impact on the adaptive immune response. Curr. Opin. Immunol., **9**, 4–9.

Miyazaki T., Matsuda Y., Toyonaga T., Mayazaki J., Yazaki Y. and Yamamura K. (1992): Prevention of autoimmune insulitis in non-obese diabetic mice by expression of major histocompatibility complex class-I Ld molecules. Proc. Natl. Acad. Sci. USA, **89**, 9519–9523.

Mondino A., Khoruts A. and Jenkins M. K. (1996): The anatomy of T-cell activation and tolerance. Proc. Natl. Acad. Sci. USA, **93**, 2245–2252.

Nishimoto H., Kikutani H., Yamamura K. and Kishimoto T. (1987): Prevention of autoimmune insulitis by expresion of I-E molecules in NOD mice. Nature, **328**, 432–434.

Ohashi P. S., Oehen S., Buerki K., Pircher H., Ohashi C. T., Odermatt B., Malissen B., Zinkernagel R. M. and Hengartner H. (1991): Ablation of tolerance and induction of diabetes by virus infection in viral antigen transgenic mice. Cell, **65**, 305–317.

Oldstone M. B., Nerenberg M., Southern P., Price J. and Lewicki H. (1991): Virus infection triggers insulin-dependent diabetes mellitus in a transgenic model: role of anti-self (virus) immune response. Cell, **65**, 319–331.

Pierre P., Turley S. J., Gatti E., Hull M., Meltzer J., Mirza A., Inaba K., Steinman R. M. and Mellman I. (1997): Developmental regulation of MHC class II transport in mouse dendritic cells. Nature, **388**, 787–792.

Pontesilli O., Carotenuto P., Gazda L. S., Pratt P. F. and Prowse S. J. (1987): Circulating lymphocyte populations and autoantibodies in non-obese diabetic (NOD) mice: a longitudinal study. Clin. Exp. Immunol., **70**, 84–93.

Pulendran B., Lingappa J., Kennedy M. K., Smith J., Teepe M., Rudensky A., Maliszewski C. R. and Maraskovsky E. (1997): Developmental pathways of dendritic cells *in vivo*: distinct function, phenotype, and localization of dendritic cell subsets in FLT3 ligand-treated mice. J. Immunol., **159**, 2222–2231.

Pulendran B., Smith J. L., Caspary G., Brasel K., Pettit D., Maraskovsky E. and Maliszewski C. R. (1999): Distinct dendritic cell subsets differentially regulate the class of immune response *in vivo*. Proc. Natl. Acad. Sci. USA, **96**, 1036–1041.

Pulendran B., Smith J. L., Jenkins M., Schoenborn M., Maraskovsky E. and Maliszewski C. R. (1998): Prevention of peripheral tolerance by a dendritic cell growth factor: Flt3 ligand as an adjuvant. J. Exp. Med., **188**, 2075–2085.

Quartey-Papafio R., Lund T., Chandler P., Picard J., Ozegbe P., Day S., Hutchings P. R., O'Reilly L., Kioussis D., Simpson E. and Cooke A. (1995): Aspartate at position 57 of non-obese diabetic I-A^{g7} beta-chain diminishes the spontaneous incidence of insulin-dependent diabetes--mellitus. J. Immunol., **154**, 5567–5575.

Rabinovitch A. (1994): Immunoregulatory and cytokine imbalances in the pathogensis of IDDM. Diabetes, **43**, 613–621.

Rademacher T. W., Williams P. and Dwek R. A. (1994): Agalactosyl glycoforms of IgG autoantibodies are pathogenic. Proc. Natl. Acad. Sci. USA, **91**, 6123–6127.

Rapoport M. J., Jaramillo A., Zipris D., Lazarus A. H., Serreze D. V., Leiter E. H., Cyopick P., Danska J. S. and Delovitch T. L. (1993): Interleukin 4 reverses T cell proliferative unresponsiveness and prevents the onset of diabetes in non-obese diabetic mice. J. Exp. Med., **178**, 87–99.

Ridgway W. M., Ito H., Fasso M., Yu C. and Fathman C. G. (1998): Analysis of the role of variation of major histocompatibility complex class II expression on non-obese diabetic (NOD) peripheral T cell response. J. Exp. Med., **188**, 2267–2275.

Rissoan M. C., Soumelis V., Kadowaki N., Grouard G., Briere F., Malefyt R. D. and Liu Y. L. (1999): Reciprocal control of T helper cell and dendritic cell differentiation. Science, **283**, 1183–1186.

Saravia-Fernandez F., Durant S., el Hasnaoui A., Dardenne M. and Homo-Delarche F. (1996): Environmental and experimental procedures leading to variations in the incidence of diabetes in the non-obese diabetic (NOD) mouse. Autoimmunity, **24**, 113–121.

Serreze D. V., Chapman H. D., Varnum D. S., Hanson M. S., Reifsnyder P. C., Richard S. D., Fleming S. A., Leiter E. H. and Shultz L. D. (1996): B lymphocytes are essential for the initiation of T cell-mediated autoimmune diabetes: Analysis of a new "speed congenic" stock of NOD. Ig mu(null) mice. J. Exp. Med., **184**, 2049–2053.

Serreze D. V., Fleming S. A., Chapman H. D., Richard S. D., Leiter E. H. and Tisch R. M. (1998): B lymphocytes are critical antigen-presenting cells for the initiation of T cell-mediated autoimmune diabetes in nonobese diabetic mice. J. Immunol., **161**, 3912–3918.

Serreze D. V., Gaedeke J. W. and Leiter E. H. (1993a): Hematopoietic stem-cell defects underlying abnormal macrophage development and maturation in NOD Lt mice. Defective regulation of cytokine receptors and protein-kinase-C. Proc. Acad. Natl. Sci. USA, **90**, 9625–9629.

Serreze D. V., Gaskins H. R. and Leiter E. H. (1993b): Defects in the differentiation and function of antigen presenting cells in NOD/Lt mice. J. Immunol., **150**, 2534–2543.

Serreze D. V. and Leiter E. H. (1994): Genetic and pathogenic pasis of autoimmune diabetes in NOD mice. Curr. Opin. Immunol., **6**, 900–906.

Singh B., Prange S. and Jevnikar A. M. (1998): Protective and destructive effects of microbial infection in insulin-dependent diabetes mellitus. Semin. Immunol., **10**, 79–86.

Steinman R. M. (1991): The dendritic cell system and its role in immunogenicity. Annu. Rev. Immunol., **9**, 271–296.

Takahashi K., Honeyman M. C. and Harrison L. C. (1998): Impaired yield, phenotype, and function of monocyte-derived dendritic cells in humans at risk for insulin-dependent diabetes. J. Immunol., **161**, 2629–2635.

Todd J. A., Bell J. I. and McDevitt H. O. (1987): HLA-DQ beta gene contributes to susceptibility and resistance to insulin-dependent diabetes mellitus. Nature, **329**, 599–604.

Trembleau S., Penna G., Gregori S., Chapman H. D., Serreze D. V., Magram J. and Adorini L. (1999): Pancreas-infiltrating Th1 cells and diabetes develop in IL-12-deficient non-obese diabetic mice. J. Immunol., **163**, 2960–2968.

Van Parijs L., Perez V. L. and Abbas A. K. (1998): Mechanisms of peripheral T cell tolerance. Novartis Found. Symp., **215**, 5–14.

Wicker L. S. (1997): Major histocompatibility complex-linked control of autoimmunity. J. Exp. Med., **186**, 973–975.

Wicker L. S., Miller B. J. and Mullen Y. (1986): Tranfer of autoimmune diabetes-mellitus with splenocytes from non-obese diabetic (NOD) mice. Diabetes, **35**, 855–860.

Wicker L. S., Todd J. A. and Peterson L. B. (1995): Genetic-control of autoimmune diabetes in the NOD mouse. Annu. Rev. Immunol., **13**, 179–200.

Winzler C., Rovere P., Rescigno M., Granucci F., Penna G., Adorini L., Zimmermann V. S., Davoust J. and Ricciardi-Castagnoli P. (1997): Maturation stages of mouse dendritic cells in growth factor-dependent long-term cultures. J. Exp. Med., **185**, 317–328.

Young J. W. and Steinman R. M. (1996): The hematopoietic development of dendritic cells: a distinct pathway for myeloid differentiation. Stem Cells, **14**, 376–387.

Ziegler A. G., Vardi P., Ricker A. T., Hattori M., Soeldner J. S. and Eisenbarth G. S. (1989): Radioassay determination of insulin autoantibodies in NOD mice. Correlation with increased risk of progression to overt diabetes. Diabetes, **38**, 358–363.

NEURO-ENDOCRINE-IMMUNE AXIS IN HUMAN RHEUMATOID ARTHRITIS

TSUYOSHI SAKANE and NOBORU SUZUKI

Departments of Immunology and Medicine, St. Marianna University School of Medicine, 2-16-1, Sugao, Miyamae-ku, Kawasaki, Kanagawa 216-8511, Japan

Abstract We present an overview of the role of neuro-endocrine-immune mechanisms in the pathophysiological responses of patients with rheumatoid arthritis (RA). In patients with RA, proinflammatory cytokines secreted by synovial cells provoke local inflammation in the joints and, simultaneously, initiate a systemic acute phase response. Thus, profound changes of the neuro-endocrine-immune axis could take place in the patients. Defects in the hypothalamus-pituitary--adrenal axis have been observed in patients with RA. Prolactin levels are often elevated and abnormal sex hormone levels have been described in RA patients. Defective neural regulation of inflammation involving neuropeptides at least partly plays a pathogenic role in RA. We and others have found that participants of the neuro-endocrine-immune interactions, such as hormones, neurotransmitters and neuropeptides, modulate RA synovial cell functions and that they are actually produced by, and their receptors are expressed on, cells within the inflammatory joint compartment. Thus, neuropeptides and hormones not only affect a systemic acute phase response of RA patients, but also modulate local inflammation directly in RA joints. These results suggest that defects in regulatory processes which are fundamental to RA may lie in the immune system, the nervous system, the endocrine system or the interactions of these. A better understanding of neuro-endocrine-immune interactions holds the promise of new approaches to the treatment of RA with the use of hormones, neurotransmitters, neuropeptides and/or their antagonists.

Key words: neuro-endocrine-immune interactions; rheumatoid arthritis; synovial cells; hypothalamus-pituitary-adrenal axis; inflammation.

Abbreviations used: RA – rheumatoid arthritis, MMP – matrix metalloproteinase, PRL – prolactin, CRH – Corticotropin-releasing hormone, IL – interleukin, TNF – tumor necrosis factor, CRH-BP – CRH-binding protein, DHEA – dehydroepiandrosterone, DHEAS – DHEA sulfate, SOM – somatostatin, SOMR – SOM receptor, PKA – protein kinase A, CREB – cyclic AMP responsive element binding protein, PRL – prolactin, PRLR – PRL receptor, GM-CSF – granulocyte/macrophage-colony stimulating factor, STAT – signal transduction and activation of transcription, Th – T helper, SLE – systemic lupus erythematosus, TIMP – tissue inhibitor of metalloproteinase, BRC – bromocriptine, HLA – human leu-

A. Górski et al. (eds.), Autoimmunity, 161–181.

cocyte antigen, CGRP – calcitonin gene-related peptide, VIP – vasoactive intestinal peptide, VIPR – VIP receptor, CGRPR – CGRP receptor, POMC – proopiomelanocortin, met-ENK – metionin-enkephalin, leu-ENK – leucine--enkephalin, END – endorphin.

1. INTRODUCTION

Rheumatoid arthritis (RA) is characterized by synovial membrane inflammation leading to chronic polyarticular destruction (Bresnihan, 1999). The inflamed synovium shows hyperplasia of synovial lining cells and lymphocytes, macrophages and granulocytes are infiltrated into the synovium (Kirkham et al., 1999; Youssef et al., 1998). Therefore, interactions between the synovial cells and infiltrating cells would occur in the RA synovium (el-Gabalawy et al., 1996; Ridley et al., 1990). It has been shown that synovial cells contribute to inflammatory responses by their production of proinflammatory cytokines, degrading enzymes such as matrix metalloproteinases (MMPs), and prostaglandins, all of which regulate cellular functions within the synovial compartment and cause tissue damage in patients with RA (Takeba et al., 2000; Wakisaka et al., 2000).

Organisms, including humans, respond to a variety of environmental stresses by mounting a coordinated complex series of adaptive responses involving the immune, nervous and endocrine systems. These adaptations are aimed at restoring the homeostatic balance and returning to the steady state (Klein, 1998). Each system in the immune, nervous and endocrine systems interacts with other systems to maintain the homeostatic balance. These interactions are facilitated by cytokines, hormones and neuropeptides, as well as their receptors which are endogenously expressed to the neural, immune and endocrine systems (Tomaszewska and Przekop, 1997). It is becoming clear that the neural, immune and endocrine systems also govern the synovial compartment (Jorgensen and Sany, 1994; Kuis and Heijnen, 1994).

There exist several clinical observations suggesting the involvement of the nervous system in the development and maintenance of RA lesions; RA that develops in patients who have had hemiplegia appears to have less affected the paralyzed limbs (Hamilton, 1983); and osteoarthritis and gout may preferentially affect the nonparalyzed side in hemiplegic patients (Sethi and Sequeira, 1990). Thus, it has been hypothesized that the nervous system and neuropeptides contribute to the inflammatory reactions and pathologic processes of RA. Similarly, involvement of the endocrine system for the pathologic responses of RA has been reported, including hypothalamic-pituitary-adrenal cortisol secretion (Gutierrez et al., 1999), prolactin (PRL) secretion (Neidhart et al., 1999) and the sex hormone status (Ostensen, 1999). Furthermore, studies of animal models of arthritis have shown that defects in the neuro-endocrine-immune communication contribute to the development of arthritis (Masi et al., 1999).

In this review, we will focus on the pathogenic roles of the neuro-endocrine-immune system in patients with RA.

2. HYPOTHALAMIC-PITUITARY-ADRENAL AXIS IN RA

The hypothalamic-pituitary-adrenal axis plays an important role in regulating and controlling immune responses, and dysfunction of the axis has been implicated in the pathogenesis of RA (Eijsbouts and Murphy, 1999).

Corticotropin-releasing hormone (CRH) is a major regulator of the hypothalamic-pituitary-adrenal axis and principal coordinator of the stress response (Webster et al., 1998). As in stress, hypothalamic CRH suppresses the immune system indirectly via increased adrenal glucocorticoid production and/or sympathetic system-mediated mechanisms. During inflammatory stress, the cytokines, tumor necrosis factor α (TNF-α), interleukin1 (IL-1) and IL-6 stimulate hypothalamic CRH secretion as a way of preventing the inflammatory reaction from overreacting. On the other hand, CRH receptors are present in peripheral sites of the immune system, including acute phase inflammatory cells such as neutrophils (Radulovic et al., 1999), and CRH promotes several immune functions *in vitro*, such as the induction of proliferation of rat splenocytes (Jessop et al., 1997). The direct role of CRH also appears to promote the inflammatory immune process *in vivo*; CRH is secreted locally in acute carrageenin-induced inflammation in rats and has predominantly proinflammatory effects (Webster et al., 1998); CRH is also expressed in the joints of Lewis rats with experimental arthritis (Crofford et al., 1992); *in vivo* neutralization of CRH by its specific antibody attenuates the inflammatory reactions in the rats (Giuffre et al., 1988).

In addition to production by immune cells, the peripheral nervous system, including the postganglionic sympathetic neurons and the sensory fibers type C, appears to contribute to CRH production in inflammatory sites (Webster et al., 1998). The production of CRH from the postganglionic sympathetic neurons may be responsible for the stress-induced activation of allergic/autoimmune phenomena. Indeed, Crofford et al. (1993) found that immunoreactive CRH is locally secreted in the synovium of patients with RA, suggesting that CRH functions as an autocrine and/or paracrine mediator of inflammation in humans as well.

The activity of CRH is modified by the presence of a 37 kDa binding protein (CRH-BP) (Woods et al., 1999). Woods et al. (1999) studied CRH and

CRH-BP in the synovial fluid of RA patients. They found that synovial fluid contains intact CRH-BP in molar excess to total CRH. The excess of CRH-BP may attenuate the inflammatory activity of CRH to reduce disease severity of RA patients.

Cutolo et al. (1999) assessed the hypothalamic-pituitary-adrenal axis function of sex hormone synthesis in patients with RA. They found that basal concentrations of dehydroepiandrosterone (DHEA) and its precursor, DHEA sulfate (DHEAS), which are intermediate metabolites of androgen synthesis, are significantly lower in premenopausal patients with RA than in premenopausal healthy controls. DHEA levels showed a significant negative correlation with the erythrocyte sedimentation rate, with platelet count and with the Steinbrocker class of the disease. There are several reports describing DHEA and DHEAS deficiency in patients with RA (Robinzon and Cutolo, 1999; Young et al., 1999). Collectively, it can be concluded that the abnormal androgen concentrations observed in patients with RA may support the implication of adrenal androgens in the immune/inflammatory cytokine--mediated mechanisms which are involved in the pathophysiology and clinical aspects of RA (Cutolo et al., 1999).

Gutierrez et al. (1999) have reported recently that the basal serum levels of cortisol in a RA group were not significantly different from those of a healthy control group. The hypoglycemia stimulation-specific "delta" cortisol response was significantly reduced for the 30 to 45 min interval in patients with RA compared with controls. They concluded that active RA is associated with a subtle dysfunction of the hypothalamic-pituitary-adrenal glucocorticoid function (Gutierrez et al., 1999). Nonetheless, current studies suggest partial defects in the hypothalamic-pituitary-adrenal axis. The significance of the defects on RA pathogenesis has also been elusive. It should be clarified whether abnormal function of the hypothalamic-pituitary-adrenal axis is the primary cause of the disease or the secondary event to the systemic inflammation of RA. Future studies should thus focus on the relationship between the modulated functions of the hypothalamic-pituitary-adrenal axis and the subsequent pathophysiologic responses of RA.

3. SOMATOSTATIN

Somatostatin (SOM) is a small peptide which was isolated originally from the hypothalamus and which inhibits the hypophysial release of several hormones (Brazeau et al., 1973). It is widely distributed throughout the central and peripheral nervous systems (Vale et al., 1976). SOM is described as an anti-proliferative molecule and an inhibitor of exocrine or endocrine secretion from a variety of tissues including the pancreas, the gastro-intestinal tract and the central and peripheral nervous systems (Gaudillere et al., 1997).

SOM also elicits inhibitory effects on both immune responses and inflammatory responses (Goetzl and Payan, 1984; Karalis et al., 1994). SOM inhibits immunoglobulin synthesis by human B lymphocytes (Kimata et al., 1993) and proliferation of human T lymphocytes (Payan et al., 1984). It has been reported that the anti-inflammatory actions of glucocorticoid are partly mediated by increased secretion of SOM (Karalis et al., 1995).

The inhibitory potential of SOM or its analogues is regarded to be applicable for the treatment of clinical conditions ranging from human cancers to Alzheimer's and Parkinson's diseases. Indeed, SOM has been shown to have analgesic properties in cluster headache (Sicuteri et al., 1984) and in cancer (Chrubasik et al., 1984). SOM was applied for inducing remission of arthralgia in patients with psoriatic arthritis (Matucci-Cerinic et al., 1988a) and also in patients with RA (Matucci-Cerinic et al., 1988b). All the data suggest that SOM may have anti-rheumatic effects.

3.1. SOM Regulates Synovial Cell Functions of RA Patients

We have conducted experiments using *in vitro* cell cultures to elucidate the effects of SOM on RA synovial cell functions. We first measured the proliferation of RA synovial cells stimulated with serum and/or TNF-α in the presence or absence of SOM. We found that SOM inhibits the proliferative responses of RA synovial cells and the proliferation of both purified RA fibroblast-like synovial cells and macrophage-like synovial cells.

We next turned our attention onto the effects of SOM on proinflammatory cytokine production, including IL-6 and IL-8 by RA synovial cells. RA synovial cells produced a large quantity of IL-6 and IL-8 in response to TNF-α stimulation; treatment of RA synovial cells with SOM suppressed IL-6 and IL-8 mRNA expression and the protein production significantly. However, SOM did not inhibit TNF-α and IL-1β production.

We further tested whether SOM inhibits the production of MMP, important molecules for joint destruction, by RA synovial cells. SOM treatment of the RA synovial cells significantly reduced MMP-1, MMP-2 and MMP-9 mRNA expression. In addition, SOM treatment reproducibly reduced MMP protein synthesis and their enzymatic activities. These results suggest beneficial effects of SOM on the pathological responses of RA. We have confirmed that these effects of SOM are not due to its direct cytotoxic mechanism (unpublished observation). There is an important report that SOM treatment induces apoptosis of some tumor cell types (Candi et al., 1995). Taken together, SOM would induce apoptotic cell death of RA synovial cells, thereby causing suppression of their functions (Wakisaka et al., 1998). SOM may thus be a desirable therapeutic strategy for treating patients with RA.

3.2. SOM-Producing Cells and SOM Receptor-Expressing Cells in RA Joints

Because we found that SOM reduces hyperfunctions of RA synovial cells, we next studied whether SOM is present within the affected joints of RA patients. It is especially important to clarify which cell type(s) is responsible for the SOM present within RA joints; SOM is delivered by the peripheral circulation or is actively produced by some cell types in the joints.

We found SOM mRNA expression by fibroblast-like synovial cells in patients with RA. We have confirmed that SOM protein is actually produced by the synovial cells in patients with RA. In contrast, RA synovium-infiltrating lymphocytes, RA peripheral blood lymphocytes and normal peripheral blood lymphocytes neither expressed SOM mRNA nor produced SOM peptide. Thus, it is evident that SOM produced by RA fibroblast-like synovial cells acts on synovial cells to modulate their own function.

SOMRs were identified in synovial tissues displaying histologic changes compatible with active RA using classic ligand-binding techniques, *in vitro* autoradiography and *in vivo* scintigraphy (Reubi et al., 1994; Vanhagen et al., 1994). The SOMRs are members of the seven transmembrane segment receptor superfamily and molecular cloning studies have identified 5 subtypes (Bell et al., 1995). We have characterized SOMR subtypes expressed on RA synovial cells. We found that subtypes 1 and 2 SOMR are expressed on RA fibroblast-like synovial cells. Of importance is the fact that expression of subtype 2 SOMR is up-regulated when synovial cells are stimulated with TNF-α. The results suggest the existence of an autoinhibitory circuit in the synovium, where an inhibitory signal of SOM could be augmented by enhanced SOMR expression in response to proinflammatory cytokine stimulation.

3.3. Molecular Mechanism of SOM Governing Synovial Cell Functions in Patients with RA

It has been shown that accumulation of intracellular cyclic AMP (cAMP) induces activation of the catalytic subunit of the phosphorylating enzyme, protein kinase A (PKA). Activation of PKA leads to the phosphorylation of ser-133 of cAMP-responsive element-binding protein (CREB); the phosphorylated CREB acts as a transcription factor to turn on the transcription and subsequent protein synthesis in certain cell types (Habener et al., 1990). It is reported that SOM inhibits adenylate cyclase activity in many tissues (Patel et al., 1990). Thus, it is likely that SOM inhibits adenylate cyclase activity and then cAMP accumulation, followed by deficient PKA activity in RA synovial cells (Reisine, 1983). This process may lead to deficient transcription factor CREB activity in the nucleus and reduced protein synthesis (Habener et al., 1990).

We have further found that CREB is importantly involved in the proinflammatory cytokine and MMP production by the RA synovial cells (Wakisaka et al., 2000). Indeed, we found that nuclear translocation of cytoplasmic CREB is induced by TNF-α stimulation in RA fibroblast-like synovial cells and that this translocation of CREB is inhibited by SOM treatment of the RA synovial cells. SOM thus inhibits RA synovial cell function by reducing CREB activity.

SOM analogues exert direct anti-proliferative actions in various tumor cells *in vitro* (Srikant and Shen, 1996). However, the mechanism of the anti--proliferative action may be distinct from that of RA synovial cells, because the tumor cells express SOMR 5, whereas RA synovial cells express SOMR 1 and 2. The intracellular signaling cascade of SOM in different cell types expressing a distinct SOMR subtype needs to be clarified.

Recent study has shown the involvement of cAMP and a cAMP-responsive element (CRE) in the up-regulation of IL-1β synthesis (Lorenz et al., 1995). This may be the case for the inhibition by SOM of the production of proinflammatory cytokines and MMPs by RA synovial cells; up-regulation of IL-6 and collagenase synthesis may involve CREB and CRE in the promoter/enhancer regions of the relevant genes.

3.4. Application of SOM on Arthritides

Matucci-Cerinic et al. (1995) studied the antiinflammatory effect of intra--articular SOM in experimental arthritis in rabbits. SOM treatment induced a reduction of knee joint swelling. This effect was shorter than that produced by triamcinolone acetonide; however, the antiinflammatory activity elicited by successive doses of triamcinolone acetonide declined both in extent and duration, while the effects of SOM remained unchanged for each successive treatment. They suggested that SOM exerts an antiinflammatory effect in experimental arthritis and may represent an alternative to corticosteroids for intra-articular therapy of arthritis (Matucci-Cerinic et al., 1995). Following that Coari et al. (1995) studied the effects of intra-articular injections of SOM on the arthritis of RA patients. The efficacy of SOM was evaluated by determining acute phase parameters (erythrocyte sedimentation rate and C-reactive protein), the thickness of the synovial membrane measured by ultrasound technique, and clinical assessment and telethermography. They clearly showed that the intra-articular injection of SOM was able to reduce the thickness of synovial membrane and to improve other clinical parameters in patients with RA, and thus indicated that SOM may directly reduce synovitis (Coari et al., 1995). SOM was also applied to patients with painful shoulder and athletes with joint diseases, and was found effective in both studies (Russo et al., 1997; Silveri et al., 1997). They concluded that SOM may be considered useful for the treatment of articular and tendineous phlogistic diseases. A large-scale controlled study of SOM is needed to clarify its effectiveness in patients with RA.

4. PROLACTIN

Prolactin (PRL) is a mammotropic neuropeptide produced by the pituitary and extrapituitary cells existing as several isoforms (Reber, 1993). The secretion of pituitary PRL is under hypothalamic control, and the cytokines IL-1, IL-2 and IL-6 stimulate pituitary PRL production, while interferon-γ (INF-γ) and endothelin-3 (ET-3) inhibit the production (Chikanza, 1999).

PRL exerts its effects via PRL receptors (PRLR) which exist as three isoforms. PRL regulates the reproduction, osmoregulation and behavior and has potent immunomodulatory effects (Chikanza, 1999). PRL is structurally related to members of the cytokine/hematopoietic growth factor family such as erythropoietin, granulocyte/macrophage-colony-stimulating factor (GM--CSF), growth hormone and IL-2 to IL-7. The PRLR is a member of the cytokine/hematopoietic growth factor receptor family. Interaction of PRL with PRLR activates the Jak kinases which phosphorylates latent signal transduction and activation of transcription (STAT) proteins, resulting in the activation of transcription (Chikanza, 1999).

It should be emphasized that PRL has immunoregulatory potential (Chikanza, 1999; Sabharwal et al., 1992). Activated lymphocytes produce PRL (Sabharwal et al., 1992), and not only lymphocytes but also monocytes in the circulation express PRLR (Russell et al., 1985). Moreover, PRL stimulates B cells to produce immunoglobulin and induces T cell proliferation (Gutierrez et al., 1996; Sabharwal et al., 1992). It is quite interesting that PRL counteracts the effects of corticosteroids by enhancing T helper (Th) 1 cell responses, and excessive Th1 cell response has been assigned an important pathogenic role in patients with RA (Chikanza, 1999).

Several investigators have demonstrated clear relationships between circulating PRL concentrations and incidence of autoimmune diseases, including systemic lupus erythematosus (SLE) (Jara et al., 1992; Neidhart, 1998), autoimmune thyroid diseases (Ferrai et al., 1983) and autoimmune Addison's disease (Lever and McKerron, 1984).

There are numerous reports describing elevated circulating PRL levels and its role in the pathogenesis of patients with RA (Folomeev et al., 1993; Ostensen, 1999); the plasma level of PRL has been shown to be significantly elevated in patients with RA compared with patients with osteoarthritis and osteomyelitis (Jorgensen et al., 1995; Mateo et al., 1988); PRL aggravated collagen-induced arthritis in mice when given during the immunization phase (Mattsson et al., 1992).

We have recently found accumulation of PRL-producing lymphocytes and PRLR-bearing synovial cells in RA synovial tissue (Nagafuchi et al., 1999). We also found that *in vitro* treatment with PRL induces enhanced proliferation of RA synovial cells. PRL treatment provoked excessive production of proinflammatory cytokines and tissue destructive proteolytic enzymes, MMP, by RA synovial cells. In addition, PRL inhibited the tissue inhibitor of metalloproteinase1 (TIMP-1) production by the synovial cells. Thus, total collagenase activity in the joints may be up-regulated in the case of excessive PRL secretion in the joints. The finding that PRL-producing lymphocytes accumulate in the RA synovial tissue and fibroblast-like synovial cells express PRLR supports the importance of T cell-synovial cell interactions for RA pathogenesis.

Figueroa et al. (1997) studied the immunological and clinical effects of PRL suppression in RA patients with active disease. They treated the patients for 3 months with bromocriptine (BRC), an inhibitor of PRL secretion. They concluded that BRC treatment induces a significant depression of the *in vitro* immune function in RA patients and that these changes are related to parameters of disease activity (Figueroa et al., 1998). Similarly, BRC has been beneficial in treating animal models of RA (Whyte and Williams, 1988). However, there are controversial reports regarding this issue (Dougados et al., 1988; Panai, 1995). We have studied the effects of BRC in *in vitro* culture of RA synovial cells. We found that BRC potently reduces proliferation of, and proinflammatory cytokine and MMP production by, RA synovial cells.

It is well known that the only consistent genetic association with RA is for genes encoded in the human leukocyte antigen (HLA) complex, particularly HLA-DR4 (Weyand and Goronzy, 1999). The PRL gene is in close proximity to the HLA region on the short arm of chromosome six. Thus, Brennan et al. (1996; 1997) found that there may be a linkage disequilibrium between HLA-DRB1 disease susceptibility alleles and microsatellite markers close to the PRL gene in women with RA. This suggests the possibility of extended haplotypes encoding for HLA-DRB1 susceptibility and for high PRL production, which contribute to susceptibility to RA. It is thus intriguing to compare PRL production by synovium-infiltrating lymphocytes and HLA haplotypes.

4.1. Calcitonin Gene-Related Peptide and Vasoactive Intestinal Peptide

Articular joints are innervated by nociceptive nerve fibers, which are capable of secreting vasodilatory neuropeptides, substance P and calcitonin gene-related peptide (CGRP) (Hökfelt et al., 1975). The phenomenon, called neurogenic inflammation, encompasses the inflammatory response of connective tissue and immune cells to neuropeptides, neurotransmitters and vasoactive amines (Kimball, 1990). Several studies suggest a close association between the development of arthritis and the nervous system in the joints (Wilder, 1995). Originally, substance P was reported to have proinflammatory effects on collagen-induced arthritis in rats. This is also true for patients with RA; substance P is importantly involved in the exacerbation of inflammation of the RA joints (Lotz et al., 1987). Anichini et al. (1997) assayed serum substance P in RA patients to evaluate whether neurogenic inflammation with substance P release is significant in RA. They found that the mean serum substance P level is significantly higher in RA patients than in controls, suggesting that neurogenic inflammation with substance P release may contribute significantly to the pathogenesis of RA.

CGRP is a 37-amino-acid neuropeptide derived from the calcitonin/CGRP gene by alternative RNA splicing (Amara et al., 1982) which has a potent vasodilatory property (Brain et al., 1985). It has also been shown that CGRP has an immune-modulating activity (Fox et al., 1997; Wang et al., 1992). In healthy humans, CGRP is present in the serum at low concentrations but is found to be elevated in several disease conditions, such as thyroid carcinoma, cluster headache and leukemia (Fanciullacci et al., 1995; Hillyard et al., 1979; Takami and Ito, 1992). In addition, it has been reported that CGRP and vasoactive intestinal peptide (VIP) concentrations are elevated in the synovial fluids of RA patients (Arnalich et al., 1994; Lygren et al., 1986), though their pathological significance in RA remained obscure.

Calza et al. (1998) conducted an immunocytochemical and *in situ* hybridization study of neuropeptides on rats with adjuvant arthritis. They quantitatively investigated peptide- and peptide mRNA-expression in the sensory circuit at the spinal level; 1) a decrease in substance P- and CGRP-

-immunoreactivities in dorsal root ganglia was observed 5 days after adjuvant injection, with recovery (CGRP) or even an increase (substance P) after 21 days; 2) CGRP and substance P peptide levels were increased in dorsal root ganglia after 21 days; 3) opioid peptide (enkephalin and dynorphin) and substance P mRNAs were strongly up-regulated in dorsal horn neurons after 21 days; and 4) a dramatic decrease in CGRP mRNA levels was found in motor neurons in the ventral horn after 21 days. A straightforward interpretation of the complicated results seems difficult. Nonetheless, these data indicate that peptide expression in dorsal root ganglia and the spinal cord is markedly influenced by severe inflammation with distinct and individual temporal patterns, which are also related to the severe rearrangement of joint structure during polyarthritis.

We therefore decided to study the effects of the neuropeptides on the RA synovial cell functions *in vitro*, because this is the most straightforward way to assign their pathological significance for RA. It has been shown that CGRP and substance P are costored and released together (Buck et al., 1982; Wiesenfeld-Hallin et al., 1984). Synovial tissue proper and juxta-articular bone have been shown to be innervated by substance P- and CGRP-containing nerves (Konttinen et al., 1994). In addition to substance P, CGRP has a vasodilatation effect (Brain et al., 1985), suggesting involvement of CGRP for the increase in the vascular permeability of RA lesions. Thus, it has been postulated that CGRP and substance P are associated with the pathophysiologic responses of RA. Furthermore, neutralization utilizing systemic administration of antibodies to substance P and/or CGRP has shown the alleviation of both neurogenic inflammation and arthritis (Konttinen et al., 1994). Thus, it is hypothesized that CGRP is involved in the development and/or exacerbation of inflammation, in synergy with substance P in patients with RA (Konttinen et al., 1994). Chemical denervation by the neurotoxin capsaicin (Levine et al., 1986) and surgical denervation (Ahmed et al., 1995) significantly reduce the occurrence of sensory neuropeptides, substance P and CGRP. Nevertheless, neither denervation could prevent the development of arthritis in rats. So far, it remains uncertain to what extent CGRP contributes to joint inflammation in humans as well as in rats.

Our *in vitro* study has clearly shown that CGRP and VIP inhibit proliferation of, and secretion of proinflammatory cytokines and MMP production by, RA synovial cells. Thus, the unmyelinated sensory afferent fibers may attenuate the pathological responses associated with RA through the release of CGRP. In this regard, it has been suggested that some of the sensory afferent fibers contain both substance P and CGRP, whereas the others contain CGRP alone (Konttinen et al., 1994). Our study suggests that CGRP inhibits pathological responses of RA and has rather beneficial effects on RA pathophysiology. It has been shown that CGRP inhibits bone resorption, further supporting the beneficial effects of CGRP on RA pathophysiology (D'Souza et al., 1986).

There are two subtypes of CGRP receptor (CGRPR) and VIP receptor (VIPR) reported so far. We found that subtype 1 CGRPR and subtype 2 VIPR are constitutively expressed on, and are functional in, RA fibroblast-like synovial cells. The affinity of the respective receptor to the relevant ligand is quite high by radioreceptor binding assays, suggesting the CGRP and VIP binding to the synovial cells is authentic.

This result also suggests the importance of the parasympathetic system in controlling joint inflammation through release of VIP (Hamilton, 1983). In this sense, it has been suggested that cathecholamines, mediators of the sympathetic system, exacerbate the pathologic responses of RA. Thus, the sympathetic system exacerbates, whereas the parasympathetic system attenuates the pathologic responses of RA. All the data support the importance of the two neuropeptides, CGRP and VIP, for the regulation of inflammation in RA joints.

CGRP and VIP inhibit adenylate cyclase activity in many tissues (Reber, 1993). Thus, it is likely that CGRP and VIP inhibit adenylate cyclase activity and then cAMP accumulation, followed by deficient PKA activity, as does SOM (Reber, 1993). This process may lead to the deficient transcription factor CREB activity in the nucleus (Takeba et al., 2000). Indeed, we found that nuclear translocation of cytoplasmic CREB and phosphorylation of ser-133 of the CREB are induced by TNF-α stimulation in RA fibroblast-like synovial cells; the translocation and phosphorylation of CREB are efficiently inhibited by CGRP and VIP treatment (Takeba et al., 1999).

Tanabe et al. (1996) have suggested that CGRPR stimulation reduces substance P-induced O2- production probably in a cAMP-associated fashion in neutrophils. Similar inhibitory responses may occur in the RA synovial cells. The CGRPR and VIPR have been found in activated lymphocytes and monocytes, thus it is likely that CGRP and VIP released from nerve endings also modulate functions of synovium-infiltrating lymphocytes (Ottaway, 1988; Umeda, 1992). Thus it is possible that CGRP and VIP exert their inhibitory effects on synovium-infiltrating lymphocytes as well (Ottaway, 1988; Umeda, 1992).

5. OPIOID

Opioid peptides contribute to the control of pain transmission by interacting with opioid receptors within the central nervous system (MacArthur et al., 1999). Opioid peptides are encoded by three genes: the proopiomelanocortin

(POMC) gene, the preproenkephalin gene and the prodynorphin gene (Danielson and Dores, 1999). They all give rise to precursor proteins, which are processed in a tissue-specific manner into small biologically active peptides (Danielson and Dores, 1999). Methionine-enkephalin (met-ENK) and leucine-enkephalin (leu-ENK), which have immunoregulatory effects on immune and inflammatory cells, are derived from pro-enkephalin A (Hiddinga et al., 1994; Munn and Lum, 1989). β-endorphin (END) is a neuroendocrine peptide with morphine-like effects produced by the anterior pituitary, cells of the immune system, and synovial cells. END is synthesized and processed within various types of immune cells under pathological conditions (Stein et al., 1990). Lymphocytes and other immune cells residing in inflamed tissue contain opioid peptides, which eventually lead to the inhibition of pain (Stein, 1995).

Several studies have been suggested the involvement of opioid peptides in the pathophysiologic responses of RA (Elbeialy et al., 1997; Kassimos et al., 1996). We found that END and ENK inhibited proliferation of RA synovial cells. END and ENK also inhibited proinflammatory cytokine production by the synovial cells. TNF-α and IL-1β production were profoundly reduced, whereas IL-6 and IL-8 production as marginally affected. These results suggest that END and ENK act selectively on macrophage-like synovial cells. Indeed, macrophage-like synovial cells expressed the μ type receptor of opioid peptides, whereas fibroblast-like synovial cells did not express the opioid peptide receptor. This finding is in striking contrast to CGRP, VIP and SOM, which inhibit IL-6 and IL-8, products of fibroblast-like synovial cells.

RA fibroblast-like synovial cells and macrophage-like synovial cells produce ENK and END. Thus, END and ENK act as autocrine and paracrine mediators of RA synovial cell functions. Elbeialy et al. (1997) found that plasma β-END levels in patients with severe RA were significantly lower than those in patients with mild RA. The mean serum level of β-END was also significantly lower in the RA group than that of normal controls. The depressed plasma β-END in patients with RA may be associated with the hyperactivity of RA synovial cells and excessive production of proinflammatory cytokines in the joints.

6. CONCLUSION

There have been several studies which suggest malfunctions of the neuro-endocrine-immune interactions in patients with RA. However, how the defective interactions contribute to the development of RA remains largely obscure. We found that several neuropeptides actually affect synovial cell function and,

Table 1. Neuropeptides involved in the regulation of local inflammation of RA

	Opioid	SOM	CGRP/VIP	Substance P	Prolactin
Production or secretion by	Macrophage-like synovial cells Fibroblast-like synovial cells	Fibroblast-like synovial cells	Nerve ending	Nerve ending	Infiltrating lymphocytes Macrophage-like synovial cells
Targets	Macrophage-like synovial cells	Fibroblast-like synovial cells	Fibroblast-like synovial cells	Fibroblast-like synovial cells	Macrophage-like synovial cells Fibroblast-like synovial cells
Effects	Proliferation ↓ TNF-α ↓ IL-1β ↓ MMP-9 ↓ IL-6 → IL-8 →	Proliferation ↓ IL-6 ↓ IL-8 ↓ MMP-1 ↓ MMP-2 ↓ MMP-9 ↓ TNF-α → IL-1β →	Proliferation ↓ IL-6 ↓ IL-8 ↓ MMP-2 ↓ TNF-α → IL-1β →	Proliferation ↑ IL-6 ↑ IL-8	Proliferation ↑ TNF-α ↑ IL-6 ↑ IL-8 ↑ MMP-2 ↑ MMP-3 ↑ MMP-8 ↑ MMP-9 ↑ TIPM-1 ↓

thus, aberrant expression of the neuropeptides leads to the exacerbation and/or attenuation of pathophysiologic responses in patients with RA. Table 1 summarizes the effects of the neuropeptides we have studied in patients with RA. The next step we have to do is to elucidate the precise mechanisms of the neuropeptides which affect the synovial cell function and the development of clinical application of the neuropeptides for treating patients with RA.

Acknowledgment. This study has been performed in collaboration with Drs. H. Nagafuchi, Y. Takeba (Departments of Immunology and Medicine, St. Marianna University School of Medicine), A. Kaneko, and T. Asai (Department of Orthopedic Surgery, Nagoya National Hospital). A part of the study in this review was supported by scientific research grants from the SRF foundation (Tokyo, Japan), the Science Research Promotion Funds from The Promotion and Mutual Aid Corporation for Private Schools of Japan (Tokyo, Japan) and a grant from the Uehara Memorial Foundation (Tokyo, Japan).

REFERENCES

Ahmed M., Srinivasan G. R., Theodorsson E., Schultzberg M. and Kreicbergs A. (1995): Effects of surgical denervation on substance P and calcitonin gene-related peptide in adjuvant arthritis. Peptides, **16**, 569–579.

Amara S. G., Jonas V., Rosenfeld M. G., Ong E. S. and Evans R. M. (1982): Alternative RNA processing in calcitionin gene expression generates mRNAs encoding different polypeptide products. Nature, **298**, 240–244.

Anichini M., Cesaretti S., Lepori M., Maddali Bongi S., Maresca M. and Zoppi M. (1997): Substance P in the serum of patients with rheumatoid arthritis. Rev. Rhum. Engl. E., **64**, 18–21.

Arnalich F., de Miguel E., Perez-Ayala C., Martinez M., Vazquez J. J., Gijon-Banos J. and Hernanz A. (1994): Neuropeptides and interleukin-6 in human joint inflammation: relationship between intraarticular substance P and interleukin-6 concentrations. Neurosci. Lett., **170**, 251–254.

Bell G. I., Yasuda K., Kong H., Law S. F., Raynor K. and Reisine T. (1995): Molecular biology of somatostatin receptors. Ciba Found. Symp., **190**, 65–88.

Brain S. D., Williams T. J., Tippins J. R., Morris H. R. and MacIntyre I. (1985): Calcitonin gene-related peptide is a potent vasodilator. Nature, **313**, 54–56.

Brazeau P., Vale W., Burgus R., Ling N., Butcher M., Rivier J. and Guillemin R. (1973): Hypothalamic polypeptide that inhibits the secretion of immunoreactive pituitary growth hormone. Science, **179**, 77–79.

Brennan P., Hajeer A., Ong K. R., Worthington J., John S., Thomson W., Silman A. and Ollier B. (1997): Allelic markers close to PRL are associated with HLA-DRB1 susceptibility alleles among women with rheumatoid arthritis and systemic lupus erythematosus. Arthritis Rheum., **40**, 1383–1386.

Brennan P., Ollier B., Worthington J., Hajeer A. and Silman A. (1996): Are both genetic and reproductive associations with rheumatoid arthritis linked to prolactin? Lancet, **348**, 106–109.

Bresnihan B. (1999): Pathogenesis of joint damage in rheumatoid arthritis. J. Rheumatol., **26**, 717–719.

Buck S. H., Walsh J. H., Yamamura H. I. and Burks T. F. (1982): Neuropeptides in sensory neurons. Life Sci., **30**, 1857–1866.

Calza L., Pozza M., Zanni M., Manzini C. U., Manzini E. and Hokfelt T. (1998): Peptide plasticity in primary sensory neurons and spinal cord during adjuvant-induced arthritis in the rat: an immunocytochemical and *in situ* hybridization study. Neuroscience, **82**, 575–589.

Candi E., Melino G., De Laurenzi V., Piacentini M., Guerrieri P., Spinedi A. and Knight R. A. (1995): Tamoxifen and somatostatin affect tumors by inducing apoptosis. Cancer Lett., **96**, 141–145.

Chikanza I. C. (1999): Prolactin and neuroimmunomodulation: *in vitro* and *in vivo* observations. Ann. NY Acad. Sci., **876**, 119–130.

Chrubasik J., Meynadier J., Blond S., Scherpereel P., Ackerman E., Weinstock M., Bonath K., Cramer H. and Wünsch E. (1984): Somatostatin, a potent analgesic. Lancet, **2**, 1208–1209.

Coari G., Di Franco M., Iagnocco A., Di Novi M. R., Mauceri M. T. and Ciocci A. (1995): Intra-articular somatostatin 14 reduces synovial thickness in rheumatoid arthritis: an ultrasonographic study. Int. J. Clin. Pharmacol. Res., **15**, 27–32.

Crofford L. J., Sano H., Karalis K., Friedman T. C., Epps H. R., Remmers E. F., Mathern P., Chrousos G. P. and Wilder R. L. (1993): Corticotropin-releasing hormone in synovial fluids and tissues of patients with rheumatoid arthritis and osteoarthritis. J. Immunol., **151**, 1587–1596.

Crofford L. J., Sano H., Karalis K., Webster E. L., Goldmuntz E. A., Chrousos G. P. and Wilder R. L. (1992): Local secretion of corticotropin-releasing hormone in the joints of Lewis rats with inflammatory arthritis. J. Clin. Invest., **90**, 2555–2564.

Cutolo M., Foppiani L., Prete C., Ballarino P., Sulli A., Villaggio B., Seriolo B., Giusti M. and Accardo S. (1999): Hypothalamic-pituitary-adrenocortical axis function in premenopausal women with rheumatoid arthritis not treated with glucocorticoid. J. Rheumatol., **26**, 282–288.

Danielson P. B. and Dores R. M. (1999): Molecular evolution of the opioid/orphanin gene family. Gen. Comp. Endocrinol., **113**, 169–186.

Dougados M., Duchesne L. and Amor B. (1988): Bromocriptine and cyclosporin A combination therapy in rheumatoid arthritis. Arthritis Rheum., **31**, 1333–1334.

D'Souza S. M., MacIntyre I., Girgis S. I. and Mundy G. R. (1986): Human synthetic calcitonin gene-related peptide inhibits bone resorption *in vitro*. Endocrinology, **119**, 58–61.

Eijsbouts A. M. and Murphy E. P. (1999): The role of the hypothalamic-pituitary-adrenal axis in rheumatoid arthritis. Baillieres Best Pract. Res. Clin. Rheumatol., **13**, 599–613.

Elbeialy A., Elbarbary M. and Kamel M. (1997): Peripheral beta-endorphin in rheumatoid arthritis. A correlation with the disease activity. Scand. J. Rheumatol., **26**, 88–91.

El-Gabalawy H., Canvin J., Ma G. M., van der Vieren M., Hoffman P., Gallatin M. and Wilkins J. (1996): Synovial distribution of alpha d/CD18, a novel leukointegrin. Comparison with other integrins and their ligands. Arthritis Rheum., **39**, 1913–1921.

Fanciullacci M., Alessandri M., Figini M., Geppetti P. and Michelacci S. (1995): Increase in plasma calcitonin gene-related peptide from the extracerebral circulation during nitroglycerin--induced cluster headache attack. Pain, **60**, 119–123.

Ferrai C., Boghen M., Paracchi A., Rampini P., Raiteri F., Benco R., Romussi M., Codecasa F., Mucci M. and Bianco M. (1983): Thyroid autoimmunity in hyperprolactinemic disorders. Acta Endocrinol., **104**, 35–41.

Figueroa F. E., Carrion F., Martinez M. E., Rivero S. and Mamani I. (1997): Bromocriptine induces immunological changes related to disease parameters in rheumatoid arthritis. Br. J. Rheumatol., **36**, 1022–1023.

Figueroa F., Carrion F., Martinez M. E., Rivero S., Mamani I. and Gonzalez G. (1998): Effects of bromocriptine in patients with active rheumatoid arthritis. Rev. Med. Chil., **126**, 33–41.

Folomeev M., Prokaeva T. and Nassonova V. (1993): Prolactin levels in men with SLE and RA. J. Rheumatol., **17**, 1569–1570.

Fox F. E., Kubin M., Cassin M., Niu Z., Hosoi J., Torii H., Granstein R. D., Trinchieri G. and Rook A. H. (1997): Calcitonin gene-related peptide inhibits proliferation and antigen presentation by human peripheral blood mononuclear cells: effects on B7; interleukin 10, and interleukin 12. J. Invest. Dermatol., **108**, 43–48.

Gaudillere A., Misery L., Bernard C., Souchier C., Claudy A. and Schmitt D. (1997): Presence of somatostatin in normal human epidermis. Br. J. Dermatol., **137**, 376–380.

Giuffre K. A., Udelsman R., Listwak S. and Chrousos G. P. (1988): Effects of immune neutralization of corticotropin-releasing hormone, adrenocorticotropin, and beta-endorphin in the surgically stressed rat. Endocrinology, **122**, 306–310.

Goetzl E. J. and Payan D. G. (1984): Inhibition by somatostatin of the release of mediators from human basophils and rat leukemic basophils. J. Immunol., **133**, 3255–3259.

Gutierrez M. A., Garcia M. E., Rodriguez J. A., Mardonez G., Jacobelli S. and Rivero S. (1999): Hypothalamic-pituitary-adrenal axis function in patients with active rheumatoid arthritis: a controlled study using insulin hypoglycemia stress test and prolactin stimulation. J. Rheumatol., **26**, 277–281.

Gutierrez M. A., Molina J. F., Jara L. J., Garcia C., Gutierrez-Urena S., Cuellar M. L., Gharavi A. and Espinoza L. R. (1996): Prolactin-induced immunoglobulin and autoantibody production by peripheral blood mononuclear cells from systemic lupus erythematosus and normal individuals. Int. Arch. Allergy Immunol., **109**, 229–235.

Habener J. F., Meyer T. E., Yun Y., Waeber G. and Hoeffler J. P. (1990): Characterization of a cAMP-regulated enhancer-binding protein. Metabolism, **39**, 13–16.

Hamilton S. (1983): Unilateral rheumatoid arthritis in hemiplegia. J. Can. Assoc. Radiol., **34**, 49–50.

Hiddinga H. J., Isaak D. D. and Lewis R. V. (1994): Enkephalin-containing peptides processed from proenkephalin significantly enhance the antibody-forming cell responses to antigens. J. Immunol., **152**, 3748–3759.

Hillyard C. J., Oscier D. G., Foa R., Catovsky D. and Goldman J. M. (1979): Immunoreactive calcitonin in leukaemia. Br. Med. J., **2**, 1392–1393.

Hökfelt T., Kellerth J. O., Nilsson G. and Pernow B. (1975): Experimental immunohistochemical studies on the localization and distribution of substance P in cat primary sensory neurons. Brain Res., **100**, 235–252.

Jara L. J., Gomez-Sanchez C., Silveiria L. H., Martinez-Osuna P., Vasey F. B. and Espinoza L. R. (1992): Hyperprolactinemia in systemic lupus erythematosus. Association with disease activity. Am. J. Med. Sci., **303**, 222–226.

Jessop D. S., Harbuz M. S., Snelson C. L., Dayan C. M. and Lightman S. L. (1997): An antisense oligodeoxynucleotide complementary to corticotropin-releasing hormone mRNA inhibits rat splenocyte proliferation *in vitro*. J. Neuroimmunol., **75**, 135–140.

Jorgensen C., Mazid H., Bologna C. and Sany J. (1995): Kinetics of prolactin release in rheumatoid arthritis. Clin. Exp. Rheumatol., **13**, 705–709.

Jorgensen C. and Sany J. (1994): Modulation of the immune response by the neuroendocrine axis in rheumatoid arthritis. Clin. Exp. Rheumatol., **12**, 435–441.

Karalis K., Mastorakos G., Chrousos G. P. and Tolis G. (1994): Somatostatin analogues suppress the inflammatory reaction *in vivo*. J. Clin. Invest., **93**, 2000–2006.

Karalis K., Mastorakos G., Sano H., Wilder R. L. and Chrousos G. P. (1995): Somatostatin may participate in the antiinflammatory actions of glucocorticoid. Endocrinology, **136**, 4133–4138.

Kassimos D., Choy E. H., Grossman A. B., Chikanza I. C. and Panayi G. S. (1996): Endogenous opioid tone in patients with rheumatoid arthritis. Br. J. Rheumatol., **35**, 436–440.

Kimata H., Yoshida A., Fujimoto M. and Mikawa H. (1993): Effect of vasoactive intestinal peptide, somatostatin, and substance P on spontaneous IgE and IgG4 production in atopic patients. J. Immunol., **150**, 4630–4640.

Kimball E. S. (1990): Substance P, cytokines, and arthritis. Ann. NY Acad. Sci., **594**, 293–308.

Kirkham B., Portek I., Lee C. S., Stavros B., Lenarczyk A., Lassere M. and Edmonds J. (1999): Intraarticular variability of synovial membrane histology, immunohistology, and cytokine mRNA expression in patients with rheumatoid arthritis. J. Rheumatol., **26**, 777–784.

Klein J. R. (1998): Hormone regulation of immune homeostasis: local or long distance? Biochem. Pharmacol., **56**, 1–5.

Konttinen Y. T., Kemppinen P., Segerberg M., Hukkanen M., Rees R., Santavirta S., Sorsa T., Pertovaara A. and Polak J. M. (1994): Peripheral and spinal neural mechanisms in arthritis, with particular reference to treatment of inflammation and pain. Arthritis Rheum., **37**, 965–982.

Kuis W. and Heijnen C. J. (1994): Rheumatoid arthritis and juvenile chronic arthritis: the role of the neuro-endocrine system. Clin. Exp. Rheumatol., **12**, S29–S34.

Lever E. G. and McKerron C. G. (1984): Autoimmune Addison's disease associated with hyperprolactinemia. Clin. Endocrinol., **21**, 451–457.

Levine J. D., Dardick S. J., Roizen M. F., Helms C. and Basbaum A. I. (1986): Contribution of sensory afferents and sympathetic efferents to joint injury in experimental arthritis. J. Neurosci., **6**, 3423–3429.

Lorenz J. J., Furdon P. J., Taylor J. D., Verghese M. W., Chandra G., Kost T. A., Haneline S. A., Roner L. A. and Gray J. G. (1995): A cyclic adenosine 3', 5'-monophosphate signal is required for the induction of IL-1β by TNF-α in human monocytes. J. Immunol., **155**, 836–844.

Lotz M., Carson D. A. and Vaughan J. H. (1987): Substance P activation of rheumatoid synovicytes: neural pathway in pathogenesis of arthritis. Science, **235**, 893–895.

Lygren I., Ostensen M., Burhol P. G. and Husby G. (1986): Gastrointestinal peptides in serum and synovial fluid from patients with inflammatory joint disease. Ann. Rheum. Dis., **45**, 637–640.

MacArthur L., Ren K., Pfaffenroth E., Franklin E. and Ruda M. A. (1999): Descending modulation of opioid-containing nociceptive neurons in rats with peripheral inflammation and hyperalgesia. Neuroscience, **88**, 499–506.

Masi A. T., Bijlsma J. W., Chikanza I. C., Pitzalis C. and Cutolo M. (1999): Neuroendocrine, immunologic, and microvascular systems interactions in rheumatoid arthritis: physiopathogenetic and therapeutic perspectives. Semin. Arthritis Rheum., **29**, 65–81.

Mateo L., Nolla J. M., Bonnin M. R., Navarro M. A. and Roig-Escofet D. (1988): High serum prolactin levels in men with rheumatoid arthritis. J. Rheumatol., **25**, 2077–2082.

Mattsson R., Mattsson A., Hansson I., Holmdahl R., Rook G. A. and Whyte A. (1992): Increased levels of prolactin during, but not after, the immunization with rat collagen II enhances the course of arthritis in DBA/1 mice. Autoimmunity, **18**, 349–353.

Matucci-Cerinic M., Borrelli F., Generini S., Cantelmo A., Marcucci I., Martelli F., Romagnoli P., Bacci S., Conz A., Marinelli P. and Marabini S. (1995): Somatostatin-induced modulation of inflammation in experimental arthritis. Arthritis Rheum., **38**, 1687–1693.

Matucci-Cerinic M., Lotti T., Cappugi P., Boddi V., Fattorini L. and Panconesi E. (1988a): Somatostatin treatment of psoriatic arthritis. Int. J. Dermatol., **27**, 56–58.

Matucci-Cerinic M. and Marabini S. (1988b): Somatostatin treatment for pain in rheumatoid arthritis: a double blind versus placebo study in knee involvement. Med. Sci. Res., **16**, 233–234.

Munn N. A. and Lum L. G. (1989): Immunoregulatory effects of alpha-endorphin, beta-endorphin, methionine-enkephalin, and adrenocorticotropic hormone on antitetanus toxoid antibody synthesis by human lymphocytes. Clin. Immunol. Immunopathol., **52**, 376–385.

Nagafuchi H., Suzuki N., Kaneko A., Asai T. and Sakane T. (1999): Prolactin locally produced by synovium infiltrating T lymphocytes induces excessive synovial cell functions in patients with rheumatoid arthritis. J. Rheumatol., **26**, 1890–1900.

Neidhart M. (1998): Prolactin in autoimmune diseases. Proc. Soc. Exp. Biol. Med., **217**, 408–419.

Neidhart M., Gay R. E. and Gay S. (1999): Prolactin and prolactin-like polypeptides in rheumatoid arthritis. Biomed. Pharmacother., **53**, 218–222.

Ostensen M. (1999): Sex hormones and pregnancy in rheumatoid arthritis and systemic lupus erythematosus. Ann. NY Acad. Sci., **876**, 131–144.

Ottaway C. A. (1988): Vasoactive intestinal peptide as a modulator of lymphocyte and immune function. Ann NY Acad. Sci., **527**, 486–500.

Panayi G. S. (1995): Hormonal control of rheumatoid inflammation. Br. Med. Bulletin, **51**, 462–471.

Patel Y. C., Murthy K. K., Escher E. E., Banvill D., Spiess J. and Srikant C. B. (1990): Mechanism of action of somatostatin: an overview of receptor function and studies of the molecular characterization and purification of somatostatin receptor proteins. Metabolism, **39**, 63–69.

Payan D. G., Hess C. A. and Goetzl E. J. (1984): Inhibition by somatostatin of the proliferation of T-lymphocytes and Molt-4 lymphoblasts. Cell. Immunol., **84**, 433–438.

Radulovic M., Dautzenberg F. M., Sydow S., Radulovic J. and Spiess J. (1999): Corticotropin--releasing factor receptor 1 in mouse spleen: expression after immune stimulation and identification of receptor-bearing cells. J. Immunol., **162**, 3013–3021.

Reber P. M. (1993): Prolactin and immunomodulation. Am. J. Med., **95**, 637–644.

Reisine T. (1983): Somatostatin desensitization: loss of the ability of somatostatin to inhibit cyclic AMP accumulation and adrenocorticotropin hormone release. J. Pharmacol. Exp. Ther., **229**, 14–20.

Reubi J. C., Waser B., Markusse H. M., Krenning E. P., Vanhagen M. and Laissue J. A. (1994): Vascular somatostatin receptors in synovium from patients with rheumatoid arthritis. Eur. J. Pharmacol., **271**, 371–378.

Ridley M. G., Kingsley G., Pitzalis C. and Panayi G. S. (1990): Monocyte activation in rheumatoid arthritis: evidence for *in situ* activation and differentiation in joints. Br. J. Rheumatol., **29**, 84–88.

Robinzon B. and Cutolo M. (1999): Should dehydroepiandrosterone replacement therapy be provided with glucocorticoid? Rheumatology, **38**, 488–495.

Russell D. H., Kibler R., Matrisian L., Larson D. F., Poulos B. and Magun B. E. (1985): Prolactin receptors on human T and B lymphocytes: antagonism of prolactin binding by cyclosporin. J. Immunol., **134**, 3027–3031.

Russo S., Mangrella M., Vitagliano S., Russo P. and Berrino L. (1997): Local administration of somatostatin in joint diseases in athletes. Minerva Med., **88**, 265–270.

Sabharwal P., Glaser R., Lafuse W., Varma S., Liu Q., Arkins S., Kooijman R., Kutz L., Kelley K. W. and Malarkey W. B. (1992): Prolactin synthesized and secreted by human peripheral blood mononuclear cells: an autocrine growth factor for lymphoproliferation. Proc. Natl. Acad. Sci. USA, **89**, 7713–7716.

Sethi S. and Sequeira W. (1990): Sparing effect of hemiplegia on scleroderma. Ann. Rheum. Dis., **49**, 999–1000.

Sicuteri F., Geppetti P., Marabini S. and Lembeck F. (1984): Pain relief by somatostatin in attacks of cluster headache. Pain, **18**, 359–365.

Silveri F., Lo-Barco C. and Brecciaroli D. (1997): Somatostatin in peri-arthropathies of the shoulder: clinical effectiveness and tolerability after sub-acromial administration. Clin. Ter., **148**, 75–81.

Srikant C. B. and Shen S. H. (1996): Octapeptide somatostatin analog SMS 201-995 induces translocation of intracellular PTP1C to membranes in MCF-7 human breast adenocarcinoma cells. Endocrinology, **137**, 3461–3468.

Stein C. (1995): The control of plain in peripheral tissue by opioids. N. Engl. J. Med., **332**, 1685–1690.

Stein C., Hassan A. H., Przewlocki R., Gramsch C., Peter K. and Herz A. (1990): Opioids from immunocytes interact with receptors on sensory nerves to inhibit nociception in inflammation. Proc. Natl. Acad. Sci. USA, **87**, 5835–5939.

Takami H. and Ito K. (1992): Calcitonin gene-related peptide as a tumor marker for medullary thyroid carcinoma. Int. Surg., **77**, 181–185.

Takeba Y., Suzuki N., Kaneko A., Asai T. and Sakane T. (1999): Evidence for neural regulation of inflammatory synovial cell functions by secreting calcitonin gene-related peptide and vasoactive intestinal peptide in patients with rheumatoid arthritis. Arthritis Rheum., **42**, 2418–2429.

Takeba Y., Suzuki N., Wakisaka S., Takeno M., Kaneko A., Asai T. and Sakane T. (2000): Involvement of cAMP responsive element binding protein (CREB) in the synovial cell hyperfunction in patients with rheumatoid arthritis. Clin. Exp. Rheumatol., **18**, 47–55.

Tanabe T., Otani H., Zeng X.-T., Mishima K., Ogawa R. and Inagaki C. (1996): Inhibitory effects of calcitonin gene-related peptide on substance-P-induced superoxide production in human neutrophils. Eur. J. Pharmacol., **314**, 175–183.

Tomaszewska D. and Przekop F. (1997): The immune-neuro-endocrine interactions. J. Physiol. Pharmacol., **48**, 139–158.

Umeda Y. (1992): Inhibition of immune responses by calcitonin gene-related peptide. Ann. NY Acad. Sci., **657**, 552–554.

Vale W., Ling N., Rivier J., Villarreal J., Rivier C., Douglas C. and Brown M. (1976): Anatomic and phylogenetic distribution of somatostatin. Metabolism, **25**, 1491–1494.

Vanhagen P. M., Markusse H. M., Lamberts S. W. J., Kwekkeboom D. J., Reubi J. C. and Krenning E. P. (1994): Somatostatin receptor imaging: the presence of somatostatin receptors in rheumatoid arthritis. Arthritis Rheum., **37**, 1521–1527.

Wakisaka S., Suzuki N., Nagafuchi H., Takeba Y., Kaneko A., Asai T. and Sakane T. (2000): Characterization of tissue outgrowth developed *in vitro* in patients with rheumatoid arthritis: involvement of T cells in the development of tissue outgrowth. Int. Arch. Allergy Immunol., **121**, 68–79.

Wakisaka S., Suzuki N., Takeba Y., Shimoyama Y., Nagafuchi H., Takeno M., Saito N., Yokoe T., Kaneko A., Asai T. and Sakane T. (1998): Modulation by proinflammatory cytokines of Fas/Fas ligand-mediated apoptotic cell death of synovial cells in patients with rheumatoid arthritis (RA). Clin. Exp. Immunol., **114**, 119–128.

Wang F., Millet I., Bottomly K. and Vignery A. (1992): Calcitonin gene-related peptide inhibits interleukin 2 production by murine T lymphocytes. J. Biol. Chem., **267**, 21052–21057.

Webster E. L., Torpy D. J., Elenkov I. J. and Chrousos G. P. (1998): Corticotropin-releasing hormone and inflammation. Ann. NY Acad. Sci., **840**, 21–32.

Weyand C. M. and Goronzy J. J. (1999): HLA polymorphisms and T cells in rheumatoid arthritis. Int. Rev. Immunol., **18**, 37–59.

Whyte A. and Williams R. O. (1988): Bromocriptine suppresses postpartum exacerbation of collagen-induced arthritis. Arthritis Rheum., **31**, 927–928.

Wiesenfeld-Hallin Z., Hokfelt T., Lundberg J. M., Forssmann W. G., Reinecke M., Tschopp F. A. and Fischer J. A. (1984): Immunoreactive calcitonin gene-related peptide and substance P coexist in sensory neurons in spinal cord and interact in spinal behavioral responses of the rat. Neurosci. Lett., **52**, 199–204.

Wilder R. L. (1995): Neuroendocrine-immune system interactions and autoimmunity. Annu. Rev. Immunol., **13**, 307–338.

Woods R. J., Kemp C. F., David J., Sumner I. G. and Lowry P. J. (1999): Cleavage of recombinant human corticotropin-releasing factor (CRF)-binding protein produces a 27-kilodalton fragment capable of binding CRF. J. Clin. Endocrinol. Metab., **84**, 2788–2794.

Young D. G., Skibinski G., Mason J. I. and James K. (1999): The influence of age and gender on serum dehydroepiandrosterone sulphate (DHEA-S), IL-6, IL-6 soluble receptor (IL-6 sR) and transforming growth factor beta 1 (TGF-beta1) levels in normal healthy blood donors. Clin. Exp. Immunol., **117**, 476–481.

Youssef P. P., Smeets T. J., Bresnihan B., Cunnane G., Fitzgerald O., Breedveld F. and Tak P. P. (1998): Microscopic measurement of cellular infiltration in the rheumatoid arthritis synovial membrane: a comparison of semiquantitative and quantitative analysis. Br. J. Rheumatol., **37**, 1003–1007.

THE ROLE OF T CELLS IN RHEUMATOID ARTHRITIS

CORNELIA M. WEYAND, EWA BRYL and JÖRG J. GORONZY

Division of Rheumatology, Mayo Foundation, Rochester, MN, USA

Abstract In rheumatoid arthritis (RA), T cells infiltrate into the synovial membrane where they initiate and maintain activation of macrophages and synovial fibroblasts, transforming them into tissue-destructive effector cells. The diversity of the disease process and the formation of complex lymphoid microstructures indicate that multiple T cell activation pathways are involved. This model is supported by the association of distinct disease patterns with different variants and combinations of HLA class II molecules. T cell pathology in RA, however, is not limited to the joint. Affected patients have major abnormalities in the T cell pool, with a marked contraction in T cell receptor diversity and an outgrowth of large clonal populations. Clonally expanded $CD4^+$ T cells lose expression of the CD28 molecule and gain expression of perforin and granzyme. Consequently, the functional profile of expanded $CD4^+CD28^{null}$ T cells is fundamentally changed and is shifted towards tissue-injurious capabilities. $CD4^+CD28^{null}$ T cells are particularly important in patients with extra-articular manifestations of RA, where they may have a direct role in vascular injury. Understanding the mechanisms underlying the loss of T cell diversity and the emergence of pro-inflammatory $CD4^+CD28^{null}$ T cell clonotypes may have implications for other autoimmune syndromes.

Key words: HLA; autoimmunity; cytokines; synovitis; oligoclonality; $CD4^+CD28^{null}$.

1. INTRODUCTION

Rheumatoid arthritis (RA) is a crippling disease that predominantly affects individuals in the prime of their lives. In early disease, pain and stiffness are the major manifestations, but, eventually, irreversible damage of joints, tendons and bones develops. The underlying lesion is a destructive inflammatory tissue composed of two components, infiltrating T cells and macrophages and resident synovial membrane cells, both of which play a part in the tissue damage (Harris, 1997). Stimulated macrophages produce inflammatory cytokines and metalloproteinases that directly damage the tissue and, in response to immune stimulation, synovial fibroblasts undergo profound

A. Górski et al. (eds.), Autoimmunity, 183–195.

phenotypic and functional changes and acquire the ability to erode and invade into cartilage and bone.

The prognosis of patients with RA is determined to some extent by the aggressiveness of the synovial lesion, but more so by the development of extra-articular rheumatoid disease (Myllykangas-Luosujarvi et al., 1995; Symmons et al., 1998; Turesson et al., 1999). Extra-articular RA can manifest in almost every organ system, emphasizing the systemic nature of the syndrome. It has been proposed that rheumatoid disease of the joint and of non-articular organs represent two, partially independent dimensions of RA (Weyand and Goronzy, 1999b; Weyand et al., 1998b). This concept has been suggested by the observation that genetic risk factors are particularly important for just one aspect of RA. The emerging model predicts that a shared risk factor exists that predisposes a person to both articular and extra-articular RA; additional risk determinants guide the disease towards one that involves predominantly joint inflammation or one characterized by extra-articular manifestations (Weyand and Goronzy, 1999a).

The traditional paradigm for the pathogenesis of RA assumes that the disease process is ultimately driven by antigen-specific T cells that recognize arthritogenic antigen and maintain the chronic inflammatory response (Weyand and Goronzy, 1997a). Although simplistic, this model has been very productive in guiding the investigation of RA. However, this paradigm has recently been challenged because it cannot account for many of the findings in affected patients. In this review, an attempt has been made to summarize recent data on T cell physiology in RA and to integrate these data into a new model of RA pathogenesis.

2. DISEASE-RISK GENES AND T CELL FUNCTION IN RA

Support for a central role of T cells in RA pathogenesis comes from the demonstration that the strongest genetic risk for RA is conferred by the HLA locus (Seldin et al., 1999). Indirect evidence from multiple lines of research supports the contention that the HLA-DRB1 locus has a direct involvement in the disease process (Goronzy and Weyand, 1995; Weyand and Goronzy, 1999a). In most ethnic groups and in most geographic regions around the world, HLA-DRB1 genes are nonrandomly distributed in patients with RA. HLA-DRB1*01 and *04 alleles are consistently over-represented and it has been hypothesized that the biologic effect is introduced by a defined sequence motif in amino acid positions 70-74 (Winchester and Gregersen, 1988). The possible involvement of polymorphic sites on HLA class II molecules has been interpreted as evidence that antigen selection and presentation are critical in RA. Accumulated data, however, question that the only function of RA-associated HLA-DRB1 molecules is peptide selection. In fact, there is increasing evidence that HLA-DR polymorphisms may not be central in disease initiation, considered to be the ultimate event in a pathological T cell response leading to RA. Not predicted by the peptide selection model, disease-associated HLA-DRB1 alleles differ in their potency to confer risk. HLA-DRB1*0401 has consistently been found to confer the highest degree of susceptibility (Goronzy and Weyand, 1993; Weyand et al., 1992). Alleles with a similar yet not identical sequence in the third hypervariable region of the HLA-DRB1 chain have been identified as the primary risk alleles for seronegative RA, a less aggressive disease variant (Weyand et al., 1995). Also, a gene-dose effect for HLA-DR alleles has been demonstrated in RA. Affected patients often inherit not only one, but frequently have two RA-risk genes (Weyand and Goronzy, 1994; Weyand et al., 1992). Allelic combinations have been associated with variations in disease severity, supporting the conclusion that HLA-DRB1 molecules function as progression factors and disease modulators instead of being involved in disease initiation.

The over-representation of RA-associated HLA-DRB1 alleles on both haplotypes has led to the proposal that MHC class II molecules influence RA pathogenesis primarily by selecting the T cell repertoire and not by presenting arthritogenic antigens (Goronzy et al., 1998; Weyand and Goronzy, 1997b; Weyand and Goronzy, 1999a). Experimental data confirm that the composition of the T cell receptor repertoire has a disease-specific fingerprint that is altered in individuals with RA when compared with age-matched healthy donors (Walser-Kuntz et al., 1995).

Studies of HLA class II molecules in RA have been helpful in dissecting the phenotypic heterogeneity of the disease (Weyand and Goronzy, 2000; Weyand et al., 1998b). Preferential expression of defined HLA-DR alleles in patient subsets with specific clinical characteristics has brought recognition that RA is a heterogeneous syndrome encompassing multiple different subtypes. MHC class II genotypes are currently being studied as biomarkers to separate RA phenotypes. The association of different HLA-DRB1 genes with distinct types of RA indicates that the contribution of HLA molecules in RA pathogenesis is complex and not limited to a single pathway.

3. T CELLS IN THE SYNOVIAL LESION

Tissue-eroding infiltrates in the synovial membrane are composed of T cells, B cells, macrophages, dendritic cells and synoviocytes. T cell dependence of the inflammatory reaction has been inferred from experiments that suggest antigen-specific activation of lesion T cells (Davis and Lipsky, 1998; Kohem et al., 1996), including *in situ* proliferation and clonal expansion of identical T cell receptors in distinct joints (Table 1) (Kato et al., 1997; Kurokawa et al., 1999; Rittner et al., 1997). Proof for the ultimate regulatory role of T cells in synovitis comes from T cell depletion experiments (Klimiuk et al., 1999). T cells were eliminated from the synovial tissue and the function of surviving cells was evaluated. These experiments were made possible by a novel "animal model" of RA. Synovial tissue from RA patients was implanted into severe combined immunodeficiency (SCID) mice to create synovium-SCID mouse chimeras. In the grafts, the disease process was well maintained, as determined by the ongoing production of the proinflammatory cytokines, IL-1, TNF-α, IL-6, IL-2 and IFN-γ. Also, the metalloproteinases, MMP-1 and MMP-3, were abundant in the engrafted tissue. Depletion of synovial T cells by treating the chimeras with anti-CD2 antibodies resulted in a prompt cessation of tissue IFN-γ production, followed by a sharp decline in the *in situ* production of IL-1α, TNF-α, MMP-1, and MMP-3. Also, the T cell growth factor IL-15, suspected to amplify T cell activation in the inflamed joint, was lost after the elimination of T cells. A critical role of the T cell product IFN-γ in regulating synovitis was demonstrated by reconstituting the synovium-SCID mouse chimeras with recombinant IFN-γ after they had received the T cell-depleting antibody treatment. Exogenous IFN-γ completely restored the production of proinflammatory monokines and tissue-digesting metalloproteinases.

Table 1. T cells in the synovial lesions

Evidence for T cell involvement in RA
Dominant population of tissue-infiltrating cells
Undergo clonal expansion in the tissue
Representation of identical T cell clones in different sites
Provide help in the formation of lymphoid microstructures
Disruption of synovitis following T cell depletion

Additional clues of the involvement of T cells in rheumatoid synovitis have come from studies of the lymphoid microstructures formed by tissue--invading lymphocytes (Table 2). Synovial infiltrates display discrete patterns, defining several subtypes of rheumatoid disease (Klimiuk et al., 1997): T cells, B cells and macrophages can be diffusely dispersed throughout the synovial membrane; T cells and B cells can be arranged in clusters that can generate fully developed germinal center reactions; or the synovitis can be characterized by granuloma formation. Germinal centers and granulomas are

Table 2. Multiple pathways of T cell activity in RA synovitis

T cells in follicular synovitis
Interact with B cells
Interact with interdigitating dendritic cells
Provide help for germinal center reactions
$CD8^+CD40$-ligand$^+$ T cells surround follicles
T cells in granulomatous synovitis
Interact with macrophages
Produce large amounts of IFN-γ
T cells in diffuse synovitis
Produce small amounts of IFN-γ
Do not form lymphoid microstructures

sophisticated microstructures that depend on T cell help. A particular CD8 T cell subset expressing CD40-ligand has been implicated in germinal center formation (Wagner et al., 1998b). A critical issue that remains is to determine whether the distinct types of synovitis reflect different causative antigens or derive from differences in the host response pattern to identical antigens.

4. T CELL ABNORMALITIES AND EXTRA-ARTICULAR DISEASE

RA patients have fundamental abnormalities in T cell function that are not restricted to the T cells participating in the synovial infiltrates. One aberration is the expansion of selected CD4 T cells to large clonal populations (Schmidt et al., 1996a; 1996b). CD4 oligoclonality is most predictably encountered in patients with extra-articular disease (Martens et al., 1997; Waase et al., 1996).

Extra-articular manifestations of RA shorten the life expectancy of the patient, attributable to cardiovascular complications. Vasculopathy in RA may take one of several forms, spanning from frank arteritis to accelerated atherosclerosis. Available data strongly suggest that vascular injury may be mediated by a unique T cell subset, the $CD4^+CD28^{null}$ T cells. CD28-deficient T cells were initially identified when clonally expanded populations from patients with severe RA were characterized (Goronzy et al., 1994). $CD4^+CD28^{null}$ T cells are a specialized subset of T cells, distinct from classical CD4 T cells (Table 3). $CD4^+CD28^{null}$ T cells produce large amounts of IFN-γ, even in the absence of costimulatory signals (Park et al., 1997). They persist over many years (Waase et al., 1996), possibly due to a defect in clonal down-sizing (Schirmer et al.,

Table 3. Comparison of $CD4^+CD28^+$ and $CD4^+CD28^{null}$ T cell subsets

Activity	$CD4^+CD28^+$ T cell	$CD4^+CD28^{null}$ T cell
Expression of α-β T cell receptor	+	+
Utilization of CD80/CD86	+	–
Expression of CD40-ligand	+	–
Production of large amounts of IFN-γ	(+)	+
Expression of perforin/granzyme B	–	+
Expansion to large clonal populations	–	+
Impaired apoptosis/clonal down-sizing	–	+
Autoreactivity	–	+

1998). Molecular characterization of these cells has demonstrated that defective transcription of the CD28 gene is related to the loss of two nuclear factors functioning as transcription initiation proteins (Vallejo et al., 1999; 1998). While deficient for these nuclear factors, $CD28^{null}$ T cells have gained expression of several other molecules, including perforin and granzyme B (Namekawa et al., 1998). As a consequence, their functional profile is changed and they can function as cytotoxic effector cells (Weyand et al., 1998a). It may be this cytotoxic potential that equips these cells to mediate endothelial injury and the vascular damage common in the extra-articular manifestations of RA. Support for a direct role of $CD4^+CD28^{null}$ T cells in vascular disease has come from studies describing the accumulation of $CD4^+CD28^{null}$ T cells in patients with acute coronary syndromes (Liuzzo et al., 1999). Clonally expanded $CD4^+CD28^{null}$ T cells have been isolated from the ruptured atherosclerotic plaque of patients with fatal myocardial infarction (Liuzzo et al., 2000).

The clonal outgrowth of $CD4^+CD28^{null}$ T cells breaks a principal rule of T cell physiology and raises the question of how selected T cell specificities can gain a survival advantage. Different mechanisms could apply, ranging from antigen-driven proliferation to defects in T cell down-sizing. A recent study of patients with RA has posed yet another possibility. Using random T cell receptor α-chain picking and limiting dilution analysis, frequencies for individual CD4 T cells have been estimated in the total T cell compartment. Frequencies of CD4 T cells using either a BV8 or BV5 gene segment for T cell receptor rearrangement were more than ten-fold higher in RA patients than in age-matched controls (Wagner et al., 1998a), suggesting that RA is associated with a marked contraction of the T cell receptor repertoire. In a contracted repertoire, some T cell specificities may reach sufficient size to be detected as frank clonal expansions. The frequency distribution of T cell receptor α-chains from RA patients, however, has indicated that the vast majority of CD4 T cells must have undergone proliferation, in most cases insufficient to appear as a clonally expanded population. In conclusion, $CD4^+CD28^{null}$ T cells that proliferate into large clonal populations in RA may represent just the tip of the iceberg in a T cell compartment characterized by oligoclonal T cell proliferation.

One of the intriguing questions that has developed from the data is the relationship between the loss of T cell diversity and autoimmune inflammatory disease. It could be argued that T cell repertoire contraction is a consequence of disease. Available data do not support this notion. Contraction in T cell diversity was found in patients very early in the disease, with no indication that persistent disease was associated with progressive loss of diversity (Wagner et al., 1998a). Also, lessons learned from experimental therapy in RA patients favor a primary deficiency in T cell homeostasis. Supported by the idea that RA is a sequela of antigen-specific T cell activation in the joint, therapeutic approaches were developed in the early 1990's to eliminate peripheral T cells in patients to open a window of opportunity for a repopulating pool with novel, non-disease-involved T cells. Antibody-mediated T cell depletion was successfully achieved in patients who received the monoclonal antibody Campath-1H, directed against the T cell and B cell antigen CD52 (Brett et al., 1996). Early after treatment, inflammatory scores dropped, but patients had reactivation of synovial inflammation while still experiencing profound peripheral lymphopenia (Matteson et al., 1995; Weinblatt et al., 1995). More importantly, the peripheral repertoire of CD4 T cells was massively contracted and dominant clonal T cell populations were shared between persistent synovial lesions and the peripheral pool (Finnegan and Schnitzer, 1997; Jendro et al., 1995). Thus, polyarthritis can persist in the setting of lymphopenia and only a small population of CD4 T cells is required to sustain synovitis. The most important information from these trials was that RA patients had marked difficulties in repopulating the T cell compartment. Peripheral CD4 T cell counts remained depressed to lymphopenic levels for an extended period, raising the interesting question whether RA patients have fundamental difficulties in generating and maintaining a diverse T cell compartment.

5. A NEW MODEL FOR RA: SYNOVITIS AS A CONSEQUENCE OF A CONTRACTED AND AUTOREACTIVE T CELL REPERTOIRE

The simplicity of the traditional paradigm, which considers RA as a disease caused by the recognition of a self antigen in the joint, has been appealing. The formulation of a new pathogenic model, however, has been necessitated by data that challenge such a simplistic view. Two major developments have shaped the emergence of the new pathogenic model. RA is now recognized as a heterogeneous syndrome. There is a diversity of disease patterns occurring in different patients. Enrichment of certain HLA-DRB1 alleles and their combinations have been associated with defined variants of disease. Sex genes have been implicated as disease modulators in population-based studies that have demonstrated male and female disease patterns of RA (Belghomari et al., 1999; Weyand et al., 1998c). Involvement of T cells in determining not only the onset but, more importantly, the evolution of the rheumatoid syndrome is indicated by the formation of lymphoid microstructures in the inflamed joint. Distinct T cell functions are relevant in the generation of granulomas, germinal centers or diffuse dispersed infiltrates (Table 2). More than one T cell activation pathway and more than one functional T cell subset must be involved in RA pathogenesis. Considering the heterogeneity of the disease process, it could be proposed that not one but multiple disease-causative antigens are relevant and that the primary defect leading to disease lies in the inability of the host immune system to maintain tolerance, not in the selective expansion of a few antigen-specific cells.

A novel view of autoimmunity in RA is encouraged by the finding that

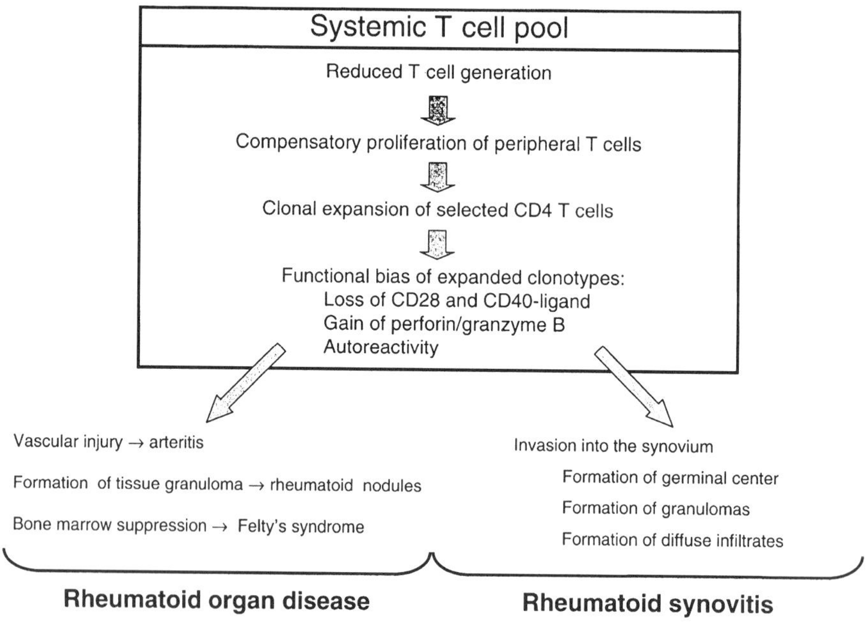

Figure 1. Hypothetical disease model for rheumatoid arthritis. At the core of rheumatoid arthritis is most likely a defect in the systemic T cell pool that leads to a clonal expansion and functional differentiation of $CD4^{+}CD28^{null}$ T cells. These cells are then able to act systemically or invade the joint, which leads to rheumatoid organ disease or rheumatoid synovitis, respectively

T cell pathology is systemic and is not limited to the joint (Fig. 1). While the perception that RA is a systemic disease fits well with clinical experience, it requires a rethinking of the simple model that tolerance is lost towards a small set of joint antigens. Rheumatoid arthritis can manifest in the lungs, the peripheral nerves, the heart and the blood vessels, creating life-threatening complications. Only a subset of patients will experience extra-articular disease, suggesting that additional genetic risk factors are necessary to superimpose nonarticular disease on synovitis. Recent findings of abnormalities in T cell homeostasis provide an opportunity to account for system-wide disease (Fig. 1). In patients with RA, the T cell pool is sharply contracted in diversity, possibly reflecting the inability to produce sufficient numbers of T cells. A defect in T cell generation would lead to clonal expansion of peripheral T cells in an attempt to fill the void. Because the dilution of autoreactive T cells may be one mechanism of maintaining tolerance, the risk of self--recognition probably increases with increasing size of individual clones. A shift of a contracted repertoire towards autoreactivity may result from other processes as well. Recognition of self-HLA-antigen complexes is possibly involved in regulating T cell survival and turnover. Replicative stress to maintain the size of the T cell compartment would increase the likelihood of anti-self-reactive T cells to emerge. Finally, it has to be considered that a higher number of self-reactive T cells could escape negative selection as the demand of the system for replenishment is increased. Experimental evidence indicates that $CD4^{+}CD28^{null}$ T cell clones isolated from RA patients are responsive to self antigens (Schmidt et al., 1996a). Their mere size could amplify their potential to cause ongoing autoimmune disease. Data have also been provided that the repertoire of naive, antigen-inexperienced T cells is biased in RA patients and that lesional T cells in the synovial infiltrates derive from T cells over-represented in the naive repertoire (Yang et al., 1999).

Why would the immune system choose the synovial membrane to display its self-reactive potential? Immune responses are not solely determined by the presence of antigen-specific precursors. Clustering of cells in time and space, surpassing of a critical mass, and signals derived from the microenvironment are all involved in making it possible for multicellular reactions to occur. Undoubtedly, the synovial microenvironment is unique and may provide necessary elements favoring the occurrence of immune reactions. Understanding the unique ingredients the joint provides may let us redirect immune responses away from the synovium. Understanding the diversity of the T cell population and stimulation pathways in RA may allow us to disrupt the inflammation with approaches that are tailored to each patient. Understanding the precise relationship between T cell homeostasis, T cell repopulation dynamics and autoreactivity may give insights that reach far beyond rheumatoid arthritis.

Acknowledgment. We thank James W. Fulbright for assistance in manuscript preparation and editing. This work was funded by grants from the National Institutes of Health (R01 AR42527 and R01 AR41974) and by the Mayo Foundation.

REFERENCES

Belghomari H., Saraux A., Allain J., Guedes C., Youinou P. and Le Goff P. (1999): Risk factors for radiographic articular destruction of hands and wrists in rheumatoid arthritis. J. Rheumatol., **26**, 2534–2538.

Brett S., Baxter G., Cooper H., Johnston J. M., Tite J. and Rapson N. (1996): Repopulation of blood lymphocyte sub-populations in rheumatoid arthritis patients treated with the depleting humanized monoclonal antibody, CAMPATH-1H. Immunology, **88**, 13–19.

Davis L. S. and Lipsky P. E. (1998): Disordered differentiation of memory T cells in rheumatoid arthritis. Rev. Rhum. Engl. Ed., **65**, 291–296.

Finnegan A. and Schnitzer T. J. (1997): Persistence of $CD4^+$ T cells in the arthritic joint after CAMPATH-1H treatment. J. Rheumatol., **24**, 1448–1449.

Goronzy J. J., Bartz-Bazzanella P., Hu W., Jendro M. C., Walser-Kuntz D. R. and Weyand C. M. (1994): Dominant clonotypes in the repertoire of peripheral $CD4^+$ T cells in rheumatoid arthritis. J. Clin. Invest., **94**, 2068–2076.

Goronzy J. J. and Weyand C. M. (1993): Interplay of T lymphocytes and HLA-DR molecules in rheumatoid arthritis. Curr. Opin. Rheumatol., **5**, 169–177.

Goronzy J. J. and Weyand C. M. (1995): T cells in rheumatoid arthritis. Paradigms and facts. Rheum. Dis. Clin. North Am., **21**, 655–674.

Goronzy J. J., Zettl A. and Weyand C. M. (1998): T cell receptor repertoire in rheumatoid arthritis. Int. Rev. Immunol., **17**, 339–363.

Harris E. D. (1997): Rheumatoid arthritis. W. B. Saunders Co., Philadelphia, 3–212.

Jendro M. C., Ganten T., Matteson E. L., Weyand C. M. and Goronzy J. J. (1995): Emergence of oligoclonal T cell populations following therapeutic T cell depletion in rheumatoid arthritis. Arthritis Rheum., **38**, 1242–1251.

Kato T., Kurokawa M., Masuko-Hongo K., Sasakawa H., Sekine T., Ueda S., Yamamoto K. and Nishioka K. (1997): T cell clonality in synovial fluid of a patient with rheumatoid arthritis: persistent but fluctuant oligoclonal T cell expansions. J. Immunol., **159**, 5143–5149.

Klimiuk P. A., Goronzy J. J., Björnsson J., Beckenbaugh R. D. and Weyand C. M. (1997): Tissue cytokine patterns distinguish variants of rheumatoid synovitis. Am. J. Pathol., **151**, 1311–1319.

Klimiuk P. A., Yang H., Goronzy J. J. and Weyand C. M. (1999): Production of cytokines and metalloproteinases in rheumatoid synovitis is T cell dependent. Clin. Immunol., **90**, 65–78.

Kohem C. L., Brezinschek R. I., Wisbey H., Tortorella C., Lipsky P. E. and Oppenheimer-Marks N. (1996): Enrichment of differentiated CD45RBdim, CD27-memory T cells in the peripheral blood, synovial fluid, and synovial tissue of patients with rheumatoid arthritis. Arthritis Rheum., **39**, 844–854.

Kurokawa M., Kato T., Masuko-Hongo K., Ueda S., Kobata T., Okubo M., Nishimaki T., Akaza T., Yoshino S., Kasukawa R., Nishioka K. and Yamamoto K. (1999): Characterisation of T cell clonotypes that accumulated in multiple joints of patients with rheumatoid arthritis. Ann. Rheum. Dis., **58**, 546–553.

Liuzzo G., Goronzy J. J., Yang H., Kopecky S. L., Holmes D. R., Frye R. L. and Weyand C. M. (2000): Monoclonal T cell prolifertation and plaque instability in acute coronary syndromes. Circulation, **101**, 2883–2888.

Liuzzo G., Kopecky S. L., Frye R. L., O'Fallon W. M., Maseri A., Goronzy J. J. and Weyand C. M. (1999): Perturbation of the T-cell repertoire in patients with unstable angina. Circulation, **100**, 2135–2139.

Martens P. B., Goronzy J. J., Schaid D. and Weyand C. M. (1997): Expansion of unusual $CD4^+$ T cells in severe rheumatoid arthritis. Arthritis Rheum., **40**, 1106–1114.

Matteson E. L., Yocum D. E., St Clair E. W., Achkar A. A., Thakor M. S., Jacobs M. R., Hays A. E., Heitman C. K. and Johnston J. M. (1995): Treatment of active refractory rheumatoid arthritis with humanized monoclonal antibody CAMPATH-1H administered by daily subcutaneous injection. Arthritis Rheum., **38**, 1187–1193.

Myllykangas-Luosujarvi R. A., Aho K. and Isomaki H. A. (1995): Mortality in rheumatoid arthritis. Semin. Arthritis Rheum., **25**, 193–202.

Namekawa T., Wagner U. G., Goronzy J. J. and Weyand C. M. (1998): Functional subsets of CD4 T cells in rheumatoid synovitis. Arthritis Rheum., **41**, 2108–2116.

Park W., Weyand C. M., Schmidt D. and Goronzy J. J. (1997): Co-stimulatory pathways controlling activation and peripheral tolerance of human $CD4^+CD28^-$ T cells. Eur. J. Immunol., **27**, 1082–1090.

Rittner H. L., Zettl A., Jendro M. C., Bartz-Bazzanella P., Goronzy J. J. and Weyand C. M. (1997): Multiple mechanisms support oligoclonal T cell expansion in rheumatoid synovitis. Mol. Med., **3**, 452–465.

Schirmer M., Vallejo A. N., Weyand C. M. and Goronzy J. J. (1998): Resistance to apoptosis and elevated expression of Bcl-2 in clonally expanded $CD4^+CD28^-$ T cells from rheumatoid arthritis patients. J. Immunol., **161**, 1018–1025.

Schmidt D., Goronzy J. J. and Weyand C. M. (1996a): $CD4^+$ $CD7^-$ $CD28^-$ T cells are expanded in rheumatoid arthritis and are characterized by autoreactivity. J. Clin. Invest., **97**, 2027–2037.

Schmidt D., Martens P. B., Weyand C. M. and Goronzy J. J. (1996b): The repertoire of $CD4^+$ $CD28^-$ T cells in rheumatoid arthritis. Mol. Med., **2**, 608–618.

Seldin M. F., Amos C. I., Ward R. and Gregersen P. K. (1999): The genetics revolution and the assault on rheumatoid arthritis. Arthritis Rheum., **42**, 1071–1079.

Symmons D. P., Jones M. A., Scott D. L. and Prior P. (1998): Longterm mortality outcome in patients with rheumatoid arthritis: early presenters continue to do well. J. Rheumatol., **25**, 1072–1077.

Turesson C., Jacobsson L. and Bergstrom U. (1999): Extra-articular rheumatoid arthritis: prevalence and mortality. Rheumatology (Oxford), **38**, 668–674.

Vallejo A. N., Brandes J. C., Weyand C. M. and Goronzy J. J. (1999): Modulation of CD28 expression: distinct regulatory pathways during activation and replicative senescence. J. Immunol., **162**, 6572–6579.

Vallejo A. N., Nestel A. R., Schirmer M., Weyand C. M. and Goronzy J. J. (1998): Aging-related deficiency of CD28 expression in $CD4^+$ T cells is associated with the loss of gene-specific nuclear factor binding activity. J. Biol. Chem., **273**, 8119–8129.

Waase I., Kayser C., Carlson P. J., Goronzy J. J. and Weyand C. M. (1996): Oligoclonal T cell proliferation in patients with rheumatoid arthritis and their unaffected siblings. Arthritis Rheum., **39**, 904–913.

Wagner U. G., Koetz K., Weyand C. M. and Goronzy J. J. (1998a): Perturbation of the T cell repertoire in rheumatoid arthritis. Proc. Natl. Acad. Sci. USA, **95**, 14447–14452.

Wagner U. G., Kurtin P. J., Wahner A., Brackertz M., Berry D. J., Goronzy J. J. and Weyand C. M. (1998b): The role of $CD8^+$ $CD40L^+$ T cells in the formation of germinal centers in rheumatoid synovitis. J. Immunol., **161**, 6390–6397.

Walser-Kuntz D. R., Weyand C. M., Weaver A. J., O'Fallon W. M. and Goronzy J. J. (1995): Mechanisms underlying the formation of the T cell receptor repertoire in rheumatoid arthritis. Immunity, **2**, 597–605.

Weinblatt M. E., Maddison P. J., Bulpitt K. J., Hazleman B. L., Urowitz M. B., Sturrock R. D., Coblyn J. S., Maier A. L., Spreen W. R. and Manna V. K. (1995): CAMPATH-1H, a humanized monoclonal antibody, in refractory rheumatoid arthritis. An intravenous dose-escalation study. Arthritis Rheum., **38**, 1589–1594.

Weyand C. M., Brandes J. C., Schmidt D., Fulbright J. W. and Goronzy J. J. (1998a): Functional properties of $CD4^+$ $CD28^-$ T cells in the aging immune system. Mech. Ageing Dev., **102**, 131–147.

Weyand C. M. and Goronzy J. J. (1994): HLA-DRB1 alleles as severity markers in RA. Bull. Rheum. Dis., **43**, 5–8.

Weyand C. M. and Goronzy J. J. (1997a): Pathogenesis of rheumatoid arthritis. Med. Clin. North Am., **81**, 29–55.

Weyand C. M. and Goronzy J. J. (1997b): The molecular basis of rheumatoid arthritis. J. Mol. Med., **75**, 772–785.

Weyand C. M. and Goronzy J. J. (1999a): HLA polymorphisms and T cells in rheumatoid arthritis. Int. Rev. Immunol., **18**, 37–59.

Weyand C. M. and Goronzy J. J. (1999b): T-cell responses in rheumatoid arthritis: systemic abnormalities-local disease. Curr. Opin. Rheumatol., **11**, 210–217.

Weyand C. M. and Goronzy J. J. (2000): HLA polymorphisms in phenotypic variants of rheumatoid arthritis. Arthritis Res., **2**, 212–216.

Weyand C. M., Hicok K. C., Conn D. L. and Goronzy J. J. (1992): The influence of HLA-DRB1 genes on disease severity in rheumatoid arthritis. Ann. Intern. Med., **117**, 801–806.

Weyand C. M., Klimiuk P. A. and Goronzy J. J. (1998b): Heterogeneity of rheumatoid arthritis: from phenotypes to genotypes. Springer Semin. Immunopathol., **20**, 5–22.

Weyand C. M., McCarthy T. G. and Goronzy J. J. (1995): Correlation between disease phenotype and genetic heterogeneity in rheumatoid arthritis. J. Clin. Invest., **95**, 2120–2126.

Weyand C. M., Schmidt D., Wagner U. and Goronzy J. J. (1998c): The influence of sex on the phenotype of rheumatoid arthritis. Arthritis Rheum., **41**, 817–822.

Winchester R. J. and Gregersen P. K. (1988): The molecular basis of susceptibility to rheumatoid arthritis: the conformational equivalence hypothesis. Springer Semin. Immunopathol., **10**, 119–139.

Yang H., Rittner H., Weyand C. M. and Goronzy J. J. (1999): Aberrations in the primary T cell receptor repertoire as a predisposition for synovial inflammation in rheumatoid arthritis. J. Invest. Med., **47**, 236–245.

INDEX